EFT Encounters with a Trapped Angel

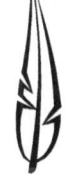

Tanya De Villiers

Encounters with a trapped angel

DEDICATION

It is my privilege and honor to dedicate this book to all those who feel trapped and contained in their own situations and circumstances. To all those who feels overlooked and not heard. Last and certainly not the least my wonderful loving family and (of course) Jamie, for their love, support and magic they bring into my life.

DISCLAIMER

EFT is a well-researched, gentle and effective way to deal with most issues in life. There is still much to be learned on many disorders and syndromes on what the effect might be of EFT as well as the possibilities. I don't advise anyone stopping therapy or seize taking their medication. Each person reading this book agrees to take full responsibility for their own health. I do advise that any self-help EFT with people or children with special needs must be done with consent and knowledge of medical/health professional.

Encounters with a trapped angel

CONTENTS

ACKNOWLEDGMENTS

Thank you to Jamie Burger and his parents for allowing me to make this journey. Many thanks to Thelma Roos for designing the Cover and Wendy Leone Cretten for the illustrations. Many special thanks to my husband, family and friends for their support. Last but not the least, to Caryl Westmore, whom has been my guiding star and support during this process.

FROM THE AUTHOR

Dear reader, thank you for taking the time to make a difference in someone's life, even if it is your own. In this book I have used many EFT scripts. Please note that these scripts are only there for your guidance. I use my intuition with each case and focus on, and study, the needs of each client. Sometimes I feel guided to use other meridian points. Feel free to explore your intuition. The main focus of this book is for you to, firstly, explore other possibilities in healing and, secondly, to open yourself to healing. Your thoughts and emotions play a huge role in where you are today and how you are feeling. Open your mind and your heart and allow the intention of love to facilitate healing. A thorough explanation on the Golden Standard EFT can be found at www.emofree.com. More information can be found at www.eftelite.com.

Encounters with a trapped angel

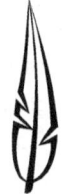

1   "AWARE, AWARE CAN I BE?"

I woke up in cold sweat... The dream was so vivid and so real. But was it real? Or was it just my twisted subconscious mind sorting herself out again? Instead of going back to sleep, I got up to make myself some coffee. It was early on Sunday morning. The bitter-sweet smell of percolated coffee filled the air and overwhelmed my senses for a moment and then, as clear as day, I knew what I needed to do. It is always amazing, that one's mind can be crystal clear for a moment, with direction and a definite purpose, and then in an instant that clarity is taken away by all the old doubts and questions.

I was thankful that my husband joined me in the kitchen and, without hesitation, I blurted out: "I want to do 30 days with Jamie". He stared at me and after a minute of silence he said; "That's great. Then you must do it". I told him about the dream I had about this beautiful trapped angel that pleaded for help. His pleadings were sincere and that was the cause of my waking up early. We sat down and started to talk the plan through on how, what and where...

My journey with this little boy began in 2011. It was a sunny morning when we attended a church service for the first time in our new community after relocating to the Western Cape from Gauteng. After the service, people came up to us, introduced themselves and welcomed us. I put on a fake smile and greeted everybody. But I was feeling angry and felt separated and almost punished by my own problems. Everything in my life was very unsettling. By nature, I am not very good at handling change so, to me, our move from Gauteng was nerve racking and very difficult. Everything was new, places, people and culture. On top of that I was facing the challenge of managing my business from 1 500km away and starting a new practice in a new city with a two-month-old baby who had developed asthma and severe colic.

I was feeling numb and disconnected from everything that was dear to me. The thought of being stuck in this numbed state scared me and I didn't know when feelings or awareness would return. On the other hand, I felt so angry that I didn't care if my feelings didn't return. What had I done wrong to deserve this? Why was I being punished? I hadn't wanted to move and I wasn't ready for the changes. And not the least of it was that my two daughters were going to grow up without grandparents or cousins around.

A very friendly woman came up to me and asked what we did and where we worked. I told her that I was a Kinder-kineticist and that I worked with children and with motor delays and special needs. I didn't want to go into details, because I really didn't want to be there. Immediately, her face lit up and she asked me if I would mind having a look at her grandson. Although I wanted to say; "No, can I please just sort out my own life first?", I looked into her eyes and I saw the same desperate need I had for help and I agreed to meet Jamie.
Jamie's grandmother introduced me to him and to the nurses at the frail-care centre of the old-age home where he was staying because there was nowhere else suitable for his care.

He was a beautiful little boy and looked so innocent, lying in his hospital bed.

But there were many things that just didn't feel right. I didn't like walking alone along the corridors to his room or seeing the forgotten and sick elderly people sitting on chairs and staring at me. I greeted them with smiles, but they said nothing and just stared at me. On top of that, I kept on forgetting how to drive to the old- age-home and the password to get in and out. My mind was too messed up.

After a few sessions of remedial therapy with Jamie, I gave up and decided to rather sort out everything over which I had control. My mind was not in a good place. I was struggling just to get up the morning and get dressed. How would I be able to sustain this masquerade of keeping up appearances and trying to perform normally? I knew that children, of any age, whether they have or don't have disorders or syndromes, could see past any mask. They intuitively sense where you are in your headspace and what your true intentions are. My decision to halt all therapy with Jamie (even if it had been only about five sessions over a period of three months) probably seemed heartless, unconsidered and selfish, but I know now that I first had to walk a special journey so that I could appreciate this ride inspired by divinity.

The flip side of the coin was that in therapy you must give a hundred percent. Anything less inhibits the child's performance, alters behavior and could very well impede a genius from reaching his or her full potential and maybe even turn to villainous acts... (Okay I am exaggerating a little - but it must be stressed that your full presence is required because children deserve it.)

As time went by I went for many courses, read many books and listened to hundreds of audio books to understand what I believed was a series of unfortunate events. I really started to feel like a professional... a professional "course-goer", that is. I had so much knowledge but didn't make the time or effort to apply it. It became part of my self-blame and punishment. I went through what I described as a "winter" in my life. Everything was dark and dry. No life or joy, no light was present. Correction - there was one light and that was the flame of my cigarette lighter that fuelled my sense of despair. I conditioned myself to procrastination and escapism. It was as if my world had been taken right out from under my feet and I had been taken to an alien land. I felt overlooked, overwhelmed, disappointed and, on top of that, very, very angry. I did not even consider, or realise then, that "my winter" had a very important purpose.

Looking back, I began to understand that the soil needed to rest so that when circumstances and the time were right, the seed that was lying there dormant could start to grow and have enough resources to start sprouting and send up shoots and even bear fruit.

After a period of time, the moping and feeling sorry for myself became unbearable. This black hole in which I was trapped became too small. I wanted to climb out, get out or give up. Having this irritating small voice inside me that was always reminding me what people would say deterred me from doing something, now unthinkable. I dug deep in our attic, searching for something that could help. Some sort of miracle cure. You know? The kind that takes five seconds and the whole world turns into rainbows and diamonds. At that stage I would have preferred a magic pill, no mess, no fuss – just add water. It was no surprise that I couldn't find anything that matched my specifications.

Once again I realised, there were only two ways to get out of a hole: 1: -someone could throw you a rope or, 2: you could climb out yourself. Seeing that I felt TOTALLY unsupported during that time I was obliged to think that I had to do this on my own. Thankfully, it was then I remembered that "Tapping Thing" or Emotional Freedom Techniques.

I first came across Emotional Freedom Techniques (EFT)

during the Tapping World Summit in 2010 and it immediately intrigued me. At that stage I didn't have any formal training in EFT and had only tried it on my own and in my own way for a short time, I felt it gave me some relief and it made sense to me, although perseverance wasn't one of my strengths at that stage. During my own dark days I completely forgot about "the Tapping Thing". It could have been that maybe I just didn't want to remember because I was too angry. I wanted to blame everything else, didn't want to take responsibility. I had started using it in my practice as a Kinder-kineticist and, as old habits die hard, I neglected to use it on myself.

In 2012 I was referred to Liesel Teversham (the author of No Problem: The Upside of Saying No) for my own private EFT session. The relief I experienced was amazing. So many things became clear. After that I decided to do the EFT Level 1 and 2 courses. It was amazing and liberating to be freed from so many emotions that were stuck in my body. I started to combine the EFT and some Brain Gym activities together with some sensory integration activities to generate results with my clients. To fulfill the winning recipe, I combined activities to activate the proprioceptors and to stimulate the communication network of the brain and nervous system. With more than 10 years' experience in Kinder-kinetics and thousands of children who had gone through my hands plus these new tools that I had acquired, I was finally ready to approach, with dedication, this little boy.

I vividly remembered the first day I brought back the CT-scan of his brain, to study it and see what the damage was. My husband and I held it to the light and before we could say anything, my four-year old daughter said without hesitation:" Ooooo, that is a beautiful brain!" I took the X-rays and placed them back into the folder, without examining them. The thoughts that rammed through my head were; "If a four-year-old can see that there is a brain who am I to argue"? That was one of the best lessons I ever learned from my daughter: The answer is sometimes right in front of you and very apparent.

Don't search for what you don't have but work with what you do have.

I quickly thought back of Dick and Ricky Hoyt, the father and disabled son who did Ironman together. Dick Hoyt and his wife were told by doctors to forget about their son and institutionalise him. But Dick said they could see in their son's eyes that he was there, present and aware. One evening, using technology to help Ricky speak, they invited friends and acquaintances to hear Ricky's first words. Much to everyone's surprise, his first words were "GO Bruins." Their journey with Ironman started with an eight kilometer fun race for people with disabilities. Ricky told his father that being in the race made him feel as if he had legs. That was enough to convince Dick that that was what they were going to do. All he had was the joy of his son and that made him to keep on swimming, cycling and running. He did it just for his son to have this experience of "no disability". The YouTube video can be seen at http://youtu.be/dDnrLv6z-mM. To what extent would we, as able-bodied people, go for a smile of appreciation or a pat on the back from a stranger?

Finally, the journey, inspired by a dream and made a reality by a five-year old boy with severe cerebral palsy was ready to begin. Today, with the greatest of gratitude, I was the divinely invited passenger who had been called to experience a lesson, or maybe lessons, that would echo for eternity.
 Within a few days of having the dream, I had to arrange for permission from his parents and from the new centre, where he was now staying, to treat him. Everything was arranged without hassles. I was ready to begin "30 days with Jamie" starting on January 21 2013.
Jamie's journey was a very different one to mine. He had not made the conscious decision to be where he was. He couldn't protest or agree. An unfortunate event had caused him to be where he was – completely dependent on people and their intentions.

On the 7th of January 2008 a healthy baby boy was born, blessing the hearts of his parents. There was great joy but also some anxiety. A few years earlier his mother had given birth to a baby boy who had, only stayed for two days and then left without announcement. Being very wary that the same would happen again, Jamie's parents guarded him like watchmen protecting a precious city.

"On the 30th of March 2009, 15-month-old Jamie Burger was rushed to the Stellenbosch Private hospital in the early hours of the morning after suffering from fever convulsions. Over the next few days, the doctors tried to bring his seizures under control and break the fever that was still spiking regularly, but to no avail. A CT scan was done which, at that stage, showed no visible damage to the brain.

However, doctors were not able to determine the cause of Jamie's illness. Due to the pressure on his brain, they could not do a lumber puncture to confirm meningitis, but were treating it as a possible cause. Blood samples were sent to laboratories to establish whether the problem was of a metabolic of nature, in view of the fact that Jamie's parents had lost their first baby to Sudden Infant Death Syndrome (SIDS) two days after being born. The private hospital pediatrician decided that it was best to have Jamie transferred to the Red Cross Children's hospital as they had not been able to bring his seizures under control and his condition was deteriorating.

Jamie was admitted to the Red Cross Children's Hospital where he immediately received the necessary treatment that the private hospital had not been able to provide. Jamie's brain activity was monitored more closely and medicine was administered to reduce the number of seizures. Another brain scan was done and this time it revealed what Jamie's parents feared most. It showed he had sustained the maximum amount of damage on both sides of the brain. Only his brain stem, which controlled his basic functions such as breathing and heartbeat, remained undamaged.

Doctors confirmed that he had, in all likelihood, lost his sight and hearing. Jamie also lost control over his muscles. This included losing control over important functions such as swallowing, easy breathing and any controlled movements such as walking or talking. Over the period that followed, Jamie's drug dosage was slowly reduced to wake him and establish whether he could cope without medical support. On first attempts it did not go well and he would stop breathing when the respiratory support system was switched off. After numerous attempts, the doctors informed Jamie's parents that they would not be putting Jamie back on breathing support and that Jamie's brain damage was so severe that they could not guarantee any life expectancy.

Jamie's parents had to prepare for the worst but, contrary to all expectations, Jamie continued to breathe on his own when the respiratory support system was switched off for the last time. In the days that followed the fever convulsions went away and his temperature, though still above normal, became more manageable. When doctors decided that Jamie was stable enough, they moved him out of ICU back to the private hospital's general pediatric ward where he remained under close supervision.

As he had lost his ability to swallow Jamie had to undergo surgery to have a gastronomy tube inserted into his stomach so that he could receive his food and medicine through the device. The operation was again followed by a difficult time with erratic spells of fever and discomfort, but Jamie managed to settle down and on the May 5 2009 Jamie left the private hospital..." – written by Stella Burger

The only place suitable to give the necessary medical care and which was willing to house Jamie was an old-age-home. He was placed in the frail- care unit. In an instant his parents' world was turned upside down. Medical expenses and care became almost unaffordable. Not only did they have to deal with the trauma of almost losing a child, followed by the distress of having a child in an almost vegetative state, but the financial burden was overwhelming. Questions of why and how consumed their lives while they urgently had to try to raise funds to pay for his care and treatment.

How difficult it must have been to be so stressed and then having to be creative in making plans to raise funds. Somehow all feelings had to be blunted in order to try to function normally and to get through. The desperately needed to be because the pain was so unbearable. Some cry, others blame but for many in a similar situation it seems like a bad dream from which they keep wishing they could wake up. Even though there are many people in the same situation at that moment, in that frame of mind, it seems as if it is only you. You are left alone in a very cold and impersonal place.

During the next few years Jamie was in and out of hospital, for various procedures. I was very excited and determined to work with this special boy. The one, who had called out to me in my sleep. Little did I know what was in store for me. Going through his background and reading the many letters from parents who had contacted me over the past year, I realised that most of the time the feeling of being overwhelmed and punished was very prevalent. It was also very difficult for the parents to come to terms with feelings of guilt and blame. . The "what ifs" and "should haves" continuously played in this movie that was, in fact, a reality.

Although I think it is necessary to start treatment or therapy as soon as possible with a child, I believe it is crucial for parents to find a method to help them to deal with these emotions. To me, the methodology in dealing with emotions is unquestionable: I use Emotional Freedom Techniques (EFT). Others might prefer different counseling or therapy. The bottom line is, however, parents must find a way to deal with their emotions.

There are many different emotions that parents go through

and many research and case studies on how EFT can very successfully help relieve stuck emotions. Once the stress has been removed from the emotions the experience of the journey could be viewed in a completely different manner. True intentions could then step forward and healing could begin. I believe children, in general, but especially those with special needs have a built-in "intention seeker". Once good intentions are present they open themselves to possibilities. Then true communication can be established and you can start to work with whatever, on that day, presents as a priority. This is when things get exciting and uplifting because you can appreciate the moment as it is; without any expectation, just acceptance and peace.

I am sending all parents in this situation love and light, and I want to tell you that you are loved and that a very wise soul has been granted to you in the form of a child. Listen to him or her with your heart and hear only love. Stand back and see the wonder.

AWAKE AND BE AWARE – Tanya de Villiers

Fatuous thoughts fondle with feeble minds,
Falling for conforming societies and colour lacking creations.
While knowing and being self-aware and awake,
is frowned upon by those threatened by truths and wonder
Distanced by prejudice, gossip and second-hand truths.

The colours are fading, so that only those really willing to see
Can create, mix and release them once more ...
Stand up brave one!!
Those willing to take responsibility for life and situation
Stand up courageous ones!!
Those willing to try to change the world for the better.
Stand up!!

Even if it is only to try...
To once again rule your world with love

Refraining from acts of fear
To walk in the footsteps of your own purpose-driven journey,
Purpose-driven day.
Rise and awake to see and really see,
What you have become, and without positive change
What you will one day be.
Awake, awake and stay aware!

The time is now and there is no more time to spare
Know your passion and your truths
Do it now,
Without delay and effort.
So healing can occur
A special gift that only you can have is so needed
To heal you, me and, of course, all of we.

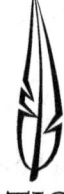

2 WHAT IS EMOTIONAL FREEDOM TECHNIQUES?

What is EFT?

Emotional Freedom Techniques (EFT) or Tapping was originally developed by Gary Craig and is often referred to as psychological acupressure. Personally, I prefer explaining it as the clearing of neurological pathways or energy blocks that inhibit healing. The technique works by releasing blockages within the energy system that cause emotional stress and discomfort. Our bodies are initially programmed to heal themselves, but because of blockages in our energy system, the natural healing patterns are interrupted. The blockages are usually caused by trauma.

Trauma is not necessarily caused by HUGE life events; it can be caused by a small but significant event. For example, a father telling his son he is stupid or not good enough or a 16-year-old boy telling a girl she is not good enough to be his girlfriend. It can be sparked by an action or words that can create a limiting belief in a person's mind and, according to that belief, he/ she will live their life.

This blockage will create emotional disharmony and it is widely accepted that emotional disharmony is the main culprit in physical symptoms and dis-ease. EFT is being accepted more and more in medical and psychiatric circles as well as in a range of psychotherapies and healing disciplines.

EFT treatment involves tapping with the fingertips on the end points of energy meridians or nerve endings that are situated just beneath the surface of the skin. The treatment is non-invasive and works on the ethos of making change as simple and as pain-free as possible.

In the short time since it was by Gary Craig in 1995, EFT has provided many people with relief from all types of conditions and problems, often in a surprisingly short time and after long and painful periods of searching for a cure or resolution. The diversity of successful treatments ranges from phobias, trauma, abuse and self-sabotaging behavioral patterns to deeply embedded emotional conditions of depression and anxiety, physical illness and addictions, to name but a few.

EFT has received attention from various healing and medical professionals; from scientists to spiritualists and many others. EFT is at the center of the rejoining of the old and new paradigms. It helps restore balance and re-awakens trust and awareness in the natural healing abilities of our minds and bodies. Using this easily applied self-help healing tool provides opportunities to achieve physical and emotional well-being in a faster time frame. This actively empowers people to contribute to their own healing and development process and facilitates a much faster relief process,

It is important to note that EFT does not discredit the medical and psychotherapeutic professions, but rather serves to contribute to a holistic healing process. It is a great tool to incorporate with other treatments.

A brief history of EFT

Rodger Callahan, an American hypnotherapist and psycho-therapist, began to develop a technique called Thought Field Therapy (TFT) in the 1980's. He came across this method by accident, when he resolved a phobia of one of his clients by following his intuition. He had been studying ancient meridian systems, which is the same system used in acupuncture. The client with whom he was working had a severe water phobia. She started to complain of feeling sick in her stomach during one of the sessions.

Callahan remembered his knowledge of the meridian system and that there was a point related to the stomach underneath the eye. As an experiment, he started tapping underneath her eye. Suddenly she jumped up, exclaimed that her phobia had gone and ran to test her fear outside at the pool. I am not sure whether she jumped in or just wet her feet – but the fact that she went near the pool and touched the water became evident that something shifted. Callahan knew he was on to something marvelous and life-changing. He started to research phobias and emotional traumas as well as their relationship to the meridians. The method was named TFT. Callahan created a series of recipes or procedures, involving various meridians, for different phobias or traumas. The procedures where extensive and very difficult to remember.

Gary Craig was one of Roger Callaghan's students. He was immediately intrigued by this method. Although TFT was very successful, Gary (being an engineer) was determined to find an easier and more user friendly way to use the method. After a lot of research, he developed EFT. This involved the same procedure being used for all disorders or traumas. EFT was introduced to the world in 1995. Since then many aspects of EFT evolved and the efficiency of EFT and the way it served the user grew dramatically. Today it is used by many professionals and much research have been done on EFT. Many, internationally renowned medical professionals, such as

Deepak Chopra, Norm Shealy and Eric Robbins, use it in their practices. Many well-known authors and public speakers, such as Jack Canfield use EFT. Bruce Lipton, a renowned molecular biologist and author, whose work can be seen on many YouTube videos, recommends EFT. Emotional wellness guru Louise Hay has recently had an EFT session with Nick Ortner and the relief and emotion she experienced on camera came as a big surprise.

The link can be found at www.youtube.com/watch?v JRfMB E2CE.

The reason for the dramatic increase in the popularity of EFT with the general public is mainly because of its high success rate. Sometimes EFT has been the only treatment that succeeded when everything else failed. I do need to emphasise that EFT is a complimentary therapy and that, in no terms, do I suggest that any other form of therapy needs to be halted. Your body knows, and, if it feels right, this might be the first place to start.

Case study 1

A slightly obese man from the Western Cape came to see me about problems he was having with relationships and communication. After a few minutes of doing EFT he revealed that he had disconnected himself from his feelings because, according to his dad, men must not show emotion. He told me his dad had said: "Things are as they are and you can't change them, no matter what emotion you have."

The belief he created was that there was no room for emotions or feelings because it wouldn't help in any case. The problems with that limiting belief were that he believed other people were not supposed to have emotions either and he was unable to connect with anyone on a deeper level. He also prevented his body from feeling anything.

> *He was completely disconnected and couldn't hear what his body either wanted or supposedly rejected. He had filled the hole within his "heart" with a lot of junk food and, in turn, he became obese.*
>
> *After a few EFT sessions he came to understand what he had been doing and he started to listen to his body and began to understand his own and other people' emotions.*

What contributes to illness and disease?

Bruce Lipton, a Molecular Biologist and author of many books explained how epigenetics works. Epigenetics is the study of changes in cellular phenotype or gene expression, caused by certain mechanisms other than changes in the underlying DNA sequence. In an experiment, he placed a single stem cell into a culture dish, where it divided every 10 hours. There were thousands of cells in the dish after two weeks. Having been taken from the same parent cell, they were all genetically identical.

He continued to divide the number of cells and placed them in three different culture dishes. The culture medium was then manipulated - equivalent to the cell's environment - in all three dishes. In one dish, the cells became bone, in another, fat, and in the last dish, muscle.

This experiment showed that the genetic pattern did not determine the cells' fate, taking in to account that the cells all had the exact same genes. It was the environment that differed. The conclusion was that if cells are in a healthy environment, they are healthy. If they're in an unhealthy environment, they become unhealthy. Lipton's argument was that moving your body from one environment to another altered the composition of the "culture medium", the blood.

Dr. Lipton further stated that the body's culture medium chemistry determined the nature of the cell's environment within you. In simpler terms, the chemistry of the blood is mostly affected by the chemicals emitted from your brain. It has been proved that brain chemistry directly adjusts the composition of the blood based upon your perceptions of life.

This means that your perception, at any moment, can influence the brain chemistry and directly affect or alter the environment of your cells and control their fate. This, in turn, means if you can alter your perception or state of mind you can directly and significantly change the fate of you cells. There are, according to Dr. Lipton, two other factors, other than the mind, which have an impact on the cells. They are toxins and trauma.

How and why EFT works?

Gary Craig explains it beautifully on one of his videos that can be found at http://www.emofree.com/eft/whatiseft.html

Perceptions and limiting beliefs can effectively be relieved by EFT, as can addictions and hereditary behaviors. The art in this therapy is to look at yourself as another person and try to see what others perceive.

There are, however, a few very important aspects that I would like you to consider.

1)   Start the process to love yourself (it might take time). You can help the process by imagining that you love yourself, loving yourself can truly change everything.

2) Consider the fact that your decision determines you destiny.

3) Open yourself to the possibility that healing and letting go might be easier than you think.

If one of the above mentioned aspects gives you a funny feeling. A feeling that you couldn't even consider doing or just doesn't feel true, that illustrates that you might have a limiting belief.

Case study 2

A very successful woman came to me for an EFT session. One of her problems was that her life was very complicated. She said she had tried everything and had spent a small fortune on trying to sort out all the disorganised files in her head. After about 15 minutes of talking and trying to determine what the focus of the session must, I suddenly realised the cause. She had a very strong belief that her life was too complicated to sort out and that nothing would work.

When I asked her if that might be the case, she started to laugh and admitted that it was. We did an EFT sequence on not being open to healing and we continued with an EFT sequence about how EFT wouldn't be able to cure this mess, because her life was so complicated. She laughed all the way through the session and kept on shaking her head. I actually started to worry. After the session we had a brief discussion and her intensity level came down considerately. I asked her why she had laughed all the way through. She exclaimed very excitedly: "I couldn't believe I had wasted all that money on therapy and I never realised I didn't want to heal."

Over the next few weeks her health increased drastically as did her mental state. She became open to the possibility that healing was easier than she thought and that her life wasn't as complicated as she had made it.

EFT unblocks stuck energy that inhibits the body from healing. It is a gentle, non-intrusive method and can be used on anyone of any age. The youngest client I have worked on was five-month- old baby. Children let go very easily, especially because they don't yet have many limiting beliefs...

We have meridians, or energy pathways, all over our bodies and one theory is that if we were to set intentions while playing sports we might have been able to resolve many issues. Take for example someone gong for a run because they feel angry or frustrated, most of the time the intention they have set before running was successful and the goal of running has been met.

The truth of the matter is that most of our lives are lived unconsciously and we let life just happen to us. The reality is: "Life isn't happening to you, but it is responding to you".
Dr. Lipton states that "The main function of the mind is to create a balance or resonance between our beliefs and the reality we experience."

How to tap?

Karate chop: (KC) On the side of the hand, halfway between the knuckle of the pinky and the wrist.
To tap you use two fingers of one hand, usually the index finger and the middle finger. To make sure you hit the right spot you can add the ring finger as well.

Eyebrow point (EB): A point situated between the nose and the beginning of the eyebrow.

Side of the Eye (SE): In the corner of the eye on the eye socket

Under the Eye (UE): in the middle of the eye on the bottom of the eye socket and beginning of the cheekbone.

Under the nose (UN): Directly underneath the nose above the upper lip.
Chin point (CP): Under the bottom lip in the middle of the chin.

Collarbone (CB): At the beginning of the collarbone.

Under the arm (UA): About four fingers under the arm, in line with the nipple (for men), and for woman it is typically in the middle of the bra strap under the arm.

Top of the head (TH): On the crown of the head.

Meridian Tapping Points

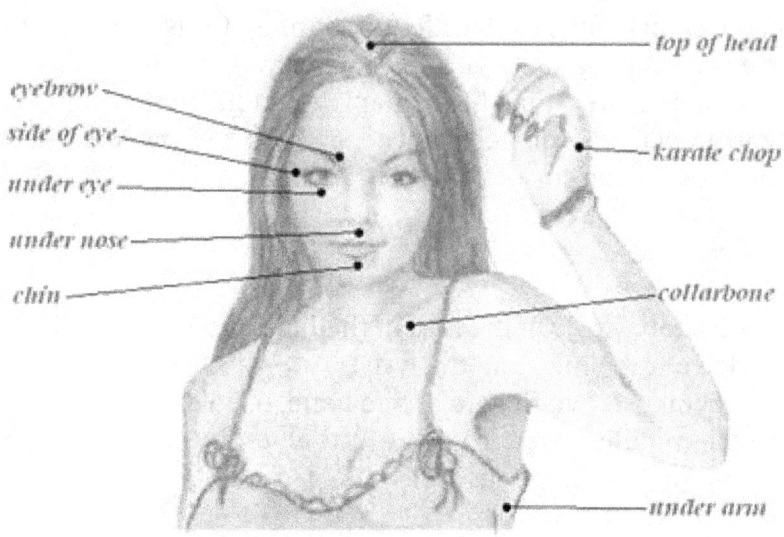

(Illustration done by Wendy Leone Cretten)

Decide on an emotion or feeling that you are experiencing or any dis-ease you feel in the body. Then determine its intensity. We usually use a scale from 0 to 10. Zero is no intensity and 10 is the highest intensity.

Some clients go past 10 to indicate that the intensity they are experiencing is "off the chart" high. With small children I usually ask them to show me with their hands and arms how bad or big the feeling is. I have used the subject of being overwhelmed as an example of how EFT is done.

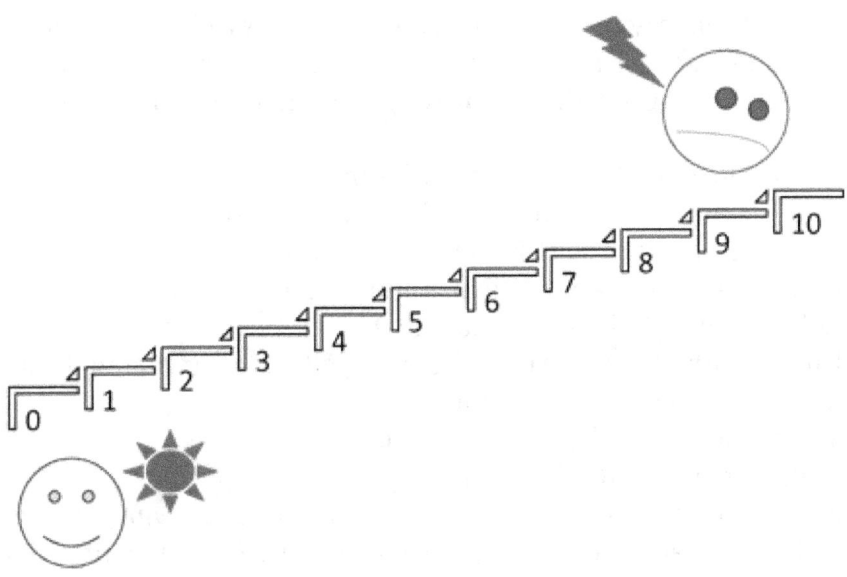

Tapping on overwhelmed (Example of surface treatment)

If you can identify the cause of this overwhelmed feeling, it will facilitate the process. I have come across many women, especially, who have this feeling of being overwhelmed. They have to perform in their careers, be good parents and wives and keep the house together, while trying to realise their own purpose for life and what makes them truly happy. This feeling of being overwhelmed drains the creative self and emphasises all the other's needs and wants. This, in turn, makes a person forget about the "me" or the self and, like a pressure cooker, the steam builds up until there is an explosion or a person begins to crumble. The following is an example of surface treatment.

Using two fingers from either hand, start to tap lightly on the karate chop (KC) point. Now say out loud "Even though I feel overwhelmed, I am in the process to love, honor and accept myself."

Remember the statement must be true. If you don't feel

comfortable saying "I love myself", change it to "I am trying to love and discover myself." Or I am in the process to love myself.
Using two, tap on the eyebrow point (EB) and say: I feel so overwhelmed.
Side of the eye (SE): All of these feelings.
Underneath the eye (UE): I don't know where to start.
Underneath the nose (UN): I feel so overwhelmed.
Chin Point (CH): I am so unsure and overwhelmed.
Collarbone (CB): How do I handle this?
Underneath the arm (UA): I am definitely overwhelmed and don't know where I must start.
Top of the head (TH): What am I going to do?
Take a deep breath and exhale.
Now scan your body for any changes. Is there any sort of feeling present, did anything else came up? Did your intensity level move up or down? You can repeat the sequence a second or a third time, until the intensity level is down.

As I mentioned in the previous chapter the parent of a child with special needs will benefit greatly from EFT. There are so many emotions to deal with. Whether or not the disorder is caused as a result of illness or trauma, birth defects, chromosomal abnormalities or anything else that might have been the cause, the screaming emotions are all the same. Children with special needs are all heart and I have learned that the moment you open your heart, true communication can begin.

Try replacing the word "overwhelmed" with any feeling that is the main focus in your life, for example feeling abandoned or misunderstood or unloved. Go through your own EFT sequence and try to determine if the intensity level is coming down or if it is shooting up. Just because you live in yourself, doesn't necessarily mean that you know yourself. It is much like being married.

People can live together for years but, because of lack of communication or the wrong kind of communication, they will have no empathy with or understanding of the other person. They might not even know what their husband or wife like or dislike.

That is how you need to work with yourself as well. Truly listen, understand and forgive, bless and love yourself, because guess what? "You are human".

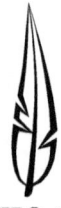

3 SETTING EYES ON AN ANGEL

Day 1, January 21, 2013

The day had arrived for my visit to Jamie and I was very nervous. I didn't really know what to expect and how he would react to the intended treatment. In my own mind I had an idea of what I intended to do, but working with children for over a decade, I was very aware that most of the time, change in a programme is inevitable.

I just hoped that I had my innovator's hat on and that creativity would fill the gaps where memory might fail me. I drove to Gabriella's centre with mixed emotions. The "Hyper-critical-me" was yelling frantically; "What have you started? Don't you have enough drama?", while the "Ever-Optimist" tried to calm the noise by humming a church choir song of some sort. I was greeted this morning by a nurse and a little boy at the gate. The boy was very friendly and presented me with a lion.

He smiled while looking down and gave a shy roar. I admired his lion and acknowledge his brave roar. He gripped my wrist tightly and walked with me to the corridor where I was supposed to meet Jamie. The pain in my wrist from his tight grip faded while I was admiring his enlightened and very genuine smile.

I thought back to my three- year stay in the United Kingdom, when I was working with children with special needs. What I have come to realize is that no matter in what country I was, the smiles of these children always managed to warm my heart. They spoke to my soul in a language that only the heart can understand.

Jamie was sitting in his chair in the corridor and I looked at the boy who was escorting me. I thought to myself: "I was just escorted by a lion...Today is going to be a Great day." I greeted Jamie in a friendly way and pushed him in his chair to the room where I would be working with him. The only room that was available to work with him was in the sleeping quarters. We were welcomed by a friendly sun painted on the wall. The thought that jumped to mind was "The Light" smiled over us and would be directing our path. Little did I know how true that thought would become.

I made some informal observations regarding Jamie's condition before I started. The observations included: Not verbal – some grunting, it sometimes seems as if he is trying to say something. Still has feeding tube in stomach. Takes nil per mouth. Chest is very bad. A lot of wheezing and an occasional attempt to cough with phlegm in the throat. "Fits" regularly. Not able to do anything that requires motor planning or motor control"

I always start with a prayer so that my intuition is switched on; because sometimes ones intuition "knows" a lot more than all of the knowledge you have accumulated over the years.
In the sessions I always try to stimulate all five senses. With

Jamie, the sense of taste was going to be a little more challenging, but definitely possible. Every session I used the same scent, called Angel Spray, so that he would begin to recognise that this was a special time. For the eyes, I used different lights, fibre optics, different coloured lights, flashlights and small lights. To stimulate the sense of hearing I would use the same "Hello" and "Good-bye" songs and use different tones of voice... The sense of touch would be stimulated during the whole session.

For the first sequence I started by stimulating the proprioceptors. (In chapter 5, I have explained this in detail). I then began with a cross crawl to try to make connection pathways and circuits for the impulses to travel along and integrating communication between the two brain hemispheres. Then I started with EFT.

KC: Even though my brain can't find my toes I love and accept myself.
EB: Where are my toes?
SE: I see them but can't feel them.
UE: Maybe I am close to discovering my toes.
UN: Then I can wiggle them.
CH: New pathways can always be formed.
CB: I can imagine feeling my toes.
UA: But I am still wondering where the feeling is in my toes.
TH: When will the toes and the brain start to communicate?
EB: Are they angry with each other?
SE: Hello there is my toes.
UE: The brain just needs to see them.
UN: They must really start to communicate.
CH: Brain please see my toes.
CB: Did the communication get lost?
UA: NO, it has only taken another path.
TH: It is in the process of discovering the toes.

Some of you might ask how I measure the intensity level. How do I know whether the intensity level came down or went up?

The truth is... I don't know... I feel and trust in my intuition. If the problem still persists it obviously means I must still work on that specific theme. It might be I must tap on something completely different, but what that is, you only start to realise as time progress.

Jamie started coughing up phlegm vigorously. I thought to myself that it could be because he was on his back for the whole 20 minutes and that made breathing a bit more difficult. My mind was busy trying to figure out how I was going to work with him if he couldn't lie on his back without coughing. "He coughed!" I suddenly realized. A proper cough. A nurse came in to see what it was that she had heard. I moved him to the recovery position and gently patted him on the back and waited a few seconds for the coughing to subside. The nurse and I looked at each other and smiled

I then started with another EFT sequence.
KC: Even though my brain can't find my feet I love and accept myself.
EB: Where are my feet?
SE: I see them but can't feel them.
UE: Maybe I am close to discovering my feet.
UN: Then I can wiggle them.
CH: New pathways can always be formed.
CB: I can imagine feeling my feet.
UA: But I am still wondering where the feeling is in my toes.
TH: When will the feet and the brain start to communicate?
EB: Are they angry with each other?
SE: Hello, there are my feet.
UE: The brain just needs to see them.
UN: They must really start to communicate.
CH: Brain please see and feel my feet.
CB: Did the communication get lost?
UA: NO, it only has taken another path.
TH: It is in the process to discover the feet.

I knew that this was going to take a lot of patience and

repetition. I then continued to just tap on his meridian points without saying anything. My leg lost feeling, because of the way I was sitting, and I had pins and needles running up and down my leg. I picked Jamie up very carefully, and placed him back into his chair. I sang the "Good-bye" song and held his hand. He seemed very relaxed when I left him. His hands, feet and legs were very relaxed and it almost seemed as if he was going to sleep. No spasms and no seizures.

My thoughts travelled far in an instant and I was again at a place of hope, peace and joy. Where suffering was a strange word that no one has ever heard of. This reminded me, if we can't dream or hope, what will there be to ignite the fires within us to do the impossible? If we can't dream or hope as opposed to denying and rejecting, nothing worthwhile would ever happen...

The session with Jamie went very well. It is strange how working with other people, will put a mirror up in front of your face. This "realisation mirror" will always reveal that which you never thought was the real problem.

Firstly, I realised I had an HUGE problem with being in the spotlight. Secondly, the confidence I thought I had, apparently disappeared between being 100 percent clear on what I must do and starting to do what I was clear about. Looking at the video footage of Day 1 I couldn't help but laugh. I was so critical about the footage: "Why was my behind in the shot the whole time? Did I really bend like that?" "I look like such an amateur." (Regardless, that I have more than 10 years' experience, and that no one has ever commented on my behind or the way I bend - or my nose or my voice.

Figure that. Who knew I was such a critic? My one and only critic. And strangely enough, one of my fears is to be in the spotlight because I don't like being criticised. What an "A-ha"-moment. Seems like it's going to be Tapping-on-Tanya tonight! LOL

Day 2. January 22, 2013

This morning Jamie had a big, beautiful smile when I greeted him. His wheezing was much better. There was no coughing and again no "fits" throughout the whole session. His hands were very relaxed and open. I picked him up with a big hug, and laid him on his bed. I started again with my usual initiation of prayer and spraying a soft sweet scent, so he would know the session was starting.

I began with a gentle massage of his feet, stimulating the nerve ends of the toes, moving to the ankles, rotating them slowly and then putting pressure on the skin next to the ankle bone. I moved to the knees bending them slowly. The knees were very stiff so I moved up to the hipbone and then down again to the knee. I used small and gentle shaking movements to help the legs relax. And they did. I pressed gently on the back of the neck, on the spine, and then tapped on the crown. I did the same with the left side of his body.

I followed with the cross crawl. Today's cross crawl was difficult and I continuously had to go back to the hip flexors to relax the legs. I then moved on to do cycling movement with the legs to keep the flow and "oil" the joints. This movement is done gently and slowly. I did the same cycling movement with the arms.

I started with the first Tapping session, doing the karate chop.
KC: Even though my body is very stiff today, I deeply and completely love and accept myself sincerely.
Even though my body is very stiff today, I am open to change and I welcome it lovingly.
EB –These legs of mine – they are so stiff. ,
SE –These legs of mine are so reluctant to change.
UE –These stubborn legs of mine.
UN –Everything is an effort.
UM –Everything is a huge effort.

CB –I am so stiff today.
UA –Why is this body fighting change?
TH –These dear, dear legs are so stiff.
EB: This dear body of mine is so special...
SE –Maybe it is resting so it can work very hard for me.
UE –These miraculous legs of mine. I might consider change.
 UN –My legs will always try to heal themselves.
CH –These legs of mine are open to positive change.
CB –These legs are open to positive change.
UA –These legs are in the process to perform optimally.
TH –These dear legs. All is well and I am peaceful and calm.

Again, many of you may ask: "Why are you talking to him and his body if you are not sure if he can comprehend or understand anything that you have just said?" Well, to me the answer is very simple... Love is an intention (not a word) that can be felt by the smallest of animals and understood by new-born babies.

Just because a baby doesn't understand the words, it doesn't mean that the intentions are lost. Therefore the energy and intentions you put into your children or work is of the upmost importance because it will resonate forever.

Case study 3

We were at a birthday party. There was a couple sitting with their five-month- old baby at our table... The baby was ill and had a fever. She didn't want to eat either. The parents of the baby were contemplating leaving because they didn't have any medicine for her fever with them. I asked the parents if we could try something before they left. We went to the baby room and sat down. I explained that I wanted to do EFT on the baby and the mother agreed. I took a few deep breaths and focused on the baby and her fever. I then started to tap on her without saying anything; I just focused on the baby and the fever. The baby was calm and watched carefully what I was doing. After a few minutes I stopped. The baby's demeanour changed completely. She was suddenly talkative and playful and her fever came down.

She started eating her yogurt. Her parents were amazed.

I went back to testing the cross crawl and Jamie's legs were very relaxed and almost felt stronger. I then continued to do EFT on the same manner as described in the previous pages, focusing on the knees. I picked him up and cradled him. I then rocked him very slowly forward and backwards to stimulate the vestibular system.

Then we started the last tapping sequence.
KC: Even though my brain can't find my legs I love and accept myself.
EB: Where are my legs?
SE: I see them but can't feel them.
UE: Maybe I am close to discovering my legs.
UN: Then I can wiggle them.
CH: New pathways can always be formed.
CB: I can imagine feeling my legs.
UA: But I am still wondering where the feeling is in my legs?
TH: When will the legs and the brain start to communicate?
EB: Are they angry with each other?
SE: Hello, there are my legs.
UE: The brain just needs to see them.
UN: They must really start to communicate.
CH: Brain please see my legs.
CB: Did the communication get lost?
UA: NO, it only has taken another path.
TH: It is in the process of discovering the legs.
I massaged his hands and thumbs to stimulate speech as explained in Brain Gym and then, giving him a big hug, I put Jamie back into his chair. With that, the session was finished. I am truly happy and grateful for the opportunity to work with him. I felt inspired and energised for some reason.
On the topic of my own insecurities of yesterday, I would say, on a scale from 1 to 10, I was on a solid 10. After a few tapping sequences last night, I was much more relaxed in front of the camera this morning. This was good because I wouldn't want external tension to influence our session.

Always remember… your intuition will NEVER fail you. You might not recognise its voice, or lack the courage or trust or "know" how to act on it. But there is NO reason in this world why your intuition will want to fail you. Listen, act and patiently watch! All is well and what an adventure that will be.

The day I recognised the inner voice.

I was busy shopping and a friend came to mind while I was looking at flowers. The thought came to me that I must buy her flowers, because she was coming over with a few other friends. Immediately I thought that the other people were going to feel left out, so I decided against it. Instead, I bought her favorite cake. That evening, when they arrived, her husband told us that it was her birthday. I felt so ashamed that I hadn't reacted to that voice, for the impact it was supposed to have on her was lost. I decided that I would never again let judgment or anticipated disappointment of others, silence the voice of wisdom.

Day 3. January 23, 2013

I was so excited about today that I couldn't wait to go. We were going to work on the eye functions. When I arrived at the centre, Jamie was still asleep in his chair. I was a little disappointed not to see the smiling boy of yesterday, but he looked very peaceful and content.

I quickly set up the room and then went to fetch him from the communal room. When I took off the belt he gave a big stretch and a yawn. I picked him up and laid him down on his bed. The Butterfly Kids CD was playing in the background. He opened his big brown eyes. The wheezing of his chest was a little worse than yesterday.

His mouth seemed dry this morning. The nurses told me he had something to drink at 6am. I asked them for an ice cube and I softly stroked it across his lips and a few small drops fell behind his lip. After the third stroke of the ice cube over his lips, he became aware of the cold and jerked his head to the side.

I apologised sincerely for the cold and it almost seemed as if a smile crept on to his face. After the "set-up procedure". Prayer and scent) we began our session, starting with massaging the feet, joints, hands, shoulders and neck. The massage was more like a stroking of the skin. There was no deep pressure, more a gentle pulling of the joints while stroking.

His right leg was very stiff today when I tried to do the cross-crawl and I had to press on the leg-buttons (as I call them) together with the hip flexors for the leg to bend. After trying numerous times, the legs were still stiff and difficult to move, so I started using EFT/Tapping. I used the scripts from yesterday and after doing it three times, I tried to work on his legs again. Now, when I tried to bend the leg the foot was pushing against my arm even harder. I got a strange feeling that this leg had nothing to do with physiology today but more with "Will-not-today-iology".

I complemented his strong kick and moved on to the next activity. I did a pre-test with eye functions, asking him to look at me, look at my finger to the right, look at my finger to the left. Look up and then down. There wasn't a very good response. I had to repeat it several times and again he could only respond to the right side.

I then started a tapping sequence: EFT on eyes
KC: Even though my I can't control my eyes or focus properly, I am in the process of teaching my body how.
EB: I can't focus.
SE: Or use my eyes properly.
UE: Maybe I am in the process of finding out how to use them.
UN: Then I can find all the beauty of life.
CH: I am struggling to see the beauty in life.
CB: There is no direction just like my eyes.
UA: I am struggling to control them.

TH: There is not much beauty that I can see.

EB: Maybe I must open myself to the possibility of seeing beautiful things.

SE: But I can't see.

UE: Can't control my eyes.

UN: They must really start to communicate.

CH: How am I going to do this?

CB: I am open and receptive to using my eyes properly.

UA: My brain will find its way to the eyes.

TH: It is in the process and I will be patient.

After three tapping sequences (I used 10 tapping points today) I asked him to look at me and he did that in an instant, the same with the left side. The right eye took a bit longer but it responded. It was amazing.

I wondered how long the effect would last. There are probably a few of you who will say it might only be a spontaneous impulse or reaction that coincidentally happened at that specific time and had nothing to do with motor planning or control, not even to mention word recognition or comprehension.

My response to that is "It MIGHT be, but it also MIGHT not be". Let us watch this space and see how the truth will reveal itself because time can only tell what limitless imagination can see. The day had arrived and I was very nervous. I didn't really know what to expect and how he would react to the purposed treatment. In my mind I had an idea of what I intended to do, but working with children for over a decade, I was under no illusion that most of the time, change in program is inevitable. I just hoped that I had my innovators hat on and that creativity would fill the gaps where memory would fail me.

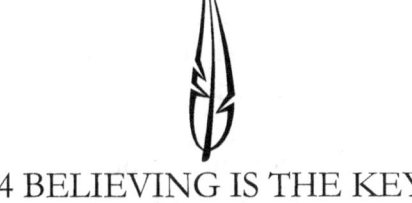

4 BELIEVING IS THE KEY

Day 4. January 24, 2013

Today was a very quiet day. The nurse opened the gate with a soft hello. The children at Gabriella's Centre were also very quiet. It reminded me vaguely of Sunday afternoons in my childhood where we children were supposed to have a quiet time and play in our rooms - probably to recharge our parents' ears for the start of the next week. Down the corridor, I could hear music playing.

Jamie was in the kitchen. "No smile today. Tanya," – I thought to myself. His bright and beautiful eyes compensated quickly for the lack of a smile. I pushed his chair to the room and picked him up and put him on his bed. His chest was wheezing. I wondered if my voice would be heard on camera over the wheezing of his chest.

The session commenced as usual, followed by the massaging and stimulation of proprioceptors. Jamie was very vocal today. He made many different noises. He lifted up his arms alternately numerous times during the massage. I kept on checking if he was having a seizure, but later I started to appreciate the spontaneous movements of his arms.

No seizure just spontaneous movements of the arms. I started to work on his left leg, but stubbornly and deliberately, he kicked his leg straight. I took the other leg and the same happened. I moved back to the left leg and with more force he kicked his leg straight when I tried to bend it. I smiled and thought: "Is Mister Jamie giving me attitude today, and not wanting to do legs? Great, I love it. A strong will can do anything if channeled in the right direction. It is, however, an art to make someone "Will" what you "Want".

The noise of his chest suddenly came to the forefront again, and I decided to give attention to that before I continued. I started the tapping sequence for his lungs and the wheezing. EFT on wheezing.

KC: Even though I can't breathe comfortably and I can't stop wheezing I lovingly accept myself and life.
EB: This wheezing.
SE: I can't breathe.
UE: I am really struggling to breath.
UN: All of the wheezing and phlegm.
CH: I can't breathe easily.
CB: I am struggling to breathe.
UA: All of this phlegm, I can't stop wheezing.
TH: Maybe I can consider taking in each breath with the greatest gratitude.
EB: Maybe I can consider that I am safe and life loves me.
SE: I trust in the process of life.
UE: I can let go of this fear of life and I take in each breath freely.
UN: Maybe I can imagine breathing freely without fear or

judgment.

CH: I can consider opening my lungs and taking in life fully.

CB: I can let go of any fear that might be present.

UA: All is well.

TH: Everything is okay, and I am safe.

During the sequences I thought, O my soul, nothing is happening. I had to quiet "that" voice and reminded myself, everything had a time. I have to let go of control. In an instant with the last tapping on the Crown Point, his wheezing subsided. Completely. He inhaled deeply and then exhaled. He was so quiet I had to make sure he was really breathing.

I was dumbstruck, even though I tried to think: "Of course this will happen with EFT," I had to swallow the tears. For the rest of the session he inhaled deeply and then exhaled. We tapped again on the eye functions and then I started with a tapping sequence of letting go of the trauma in the cell memories. The purpose of this was that the memories in the cells could assist with the healing of the body.

After the sequences, I held him on my knee and rocked him forward and backwards while singing a song. Then I put him back into the chair. What a great session!! The video can be seen on the following link: http://youtu.be/nIZAlBObeZc. The EFT script is not the same as that written in the previous page, but it is also efficient. It is important to take each person as an individual case and to listen to your heart and intuition when doing EFT. You might feel the need to tap on another meridian or place, as I have done in the video, because that is what my intuition told me. The body knows; we must listen.

Day 5. January 25, 2013

I watched the clock with great anticipation this morning. Yesterday was a crazy day and I drove a few people (sorry, my Love) up the wall, just to get the video of Day Four up and running. (I was just so excited!). One of my computers crashed while the other refused to go on to the Internet. I had to post my blog at my brother in-law's house yesterday evening. Then the saga of the video... I had phoned many people to find out how to post a video. Many of them charged an arm or a leg, which I couldn't afford.

Others tried to help me with no success. That evening friends came to visit and just before they left I mentioned the video and in less than two minutes one of my friends showed me how to do it and the video was up and running. How amazing was that? The timing was perfect. I reminded myself that sometimes I mustn't force things and work up so much emotion, relax, divine time is always the right time. I suddenly realised that my mouth was dry and wondered why it had been for the past five days every morning before I left to go to Jamie.

I made a mental note to tap on this issue when I was back at home, because I guessed there must be some tension still left or maybe some anxiousness. I left this thought with my glass of water on the counter and climbed into my car.

A very pale and not-so-happy Jamie "greeted" me in the kitchen. His energy was very low. My heart fell to my stomach, but I quickly put it back in its place to warmly and lovingly greet him with a hug and a kiss.

Louise Hay's words resonated in my head: "Today is a new day, all is well". My scientific brain immediately questioned the retention aspect and I abruptly had to silence each and every voice, opinion or theory in my head. The friendly nurse asked if she could quickly change him, before we started the session. That gave me a few minutes to gather my thoughts.

I went to Jamie's room and composed my thoughts and myself. I briefly thought of the Creation. God took seven days to create the Earth, not 1. Everything had a sequence and had to be put into place before the next day so that the next creation could take place. This is exactly the same with our lives: we must get the sequence right otherwise it might take a bit longer. For now, this thought would do, I decided.

"I let go of control, everything has a time and place." - I affirmed. The nurse carried Jamie to his bed and I positioned him comfortably. I noticed that his wheezing came back, but I knew that during the session it would get better again. (It took 10 minutes, for the wheezing to subside).

"Now let's have some fun," I said to him. I sang him a few songs while massaging and stimulating the proprioceptors. I started with rolling his shoulders and arms (first together and then alternating) and then rolling legs. The arms and legs gave some resistance and it felt a bit stronger, while his eyes honoured me countless times, with eye contact.

I started EFT, tapping on not feeling well today. He gave a huge yawn of release during this tapping sequence. I then continued tapping on letting this ,"not- so-well" feeling , go while using, again, "every day in every way I am getting better and better"- Émile Coué, (1857 1926) a French Psychologist.

I started doing the cross-crawl. During the session I kept on testing his eyes and the functioning of his arms and legs. We did tapping on "the brain not successfully communicating with my body". Looking at the video footage later I could see all the yawns and all the eye movements while tapping. It was wonderful.

Then last, but not least, the ""Good-bye" song and a big hug. My thoughts were: Tomorrow is also a new day. With faith I will look forward to it. Every blink of an eye and every smile is an absolute wonder of creation. Let's marvel at the wonders of our bodies and be grateful for all the functions that we so easily take for granted. "There must be a certain kind of darkness for us to see the stars."- Author unknown to me. I look forward to see each star and meet the sun, when it is its time to shine.

Day 6. January 26, 2013

Suddenly I realised I was staring at the ceiling and not sleeping anymore. I smiled and looked at my alarm, not even close to the jump-out-of-bed-time. "Yeah, I won!" I jokingly thought. The house was very quiet and I inhaled the silence, because I knew, in less than two hours all of this was about to change.
However, I was so excited I almost felt like waking up my family. Outside, the fresh air greeted me softly and reminded me to be grateful for each and every breath. "All is well, everything is going to be okay, and I am safe." Louise Hay reminded me again. Let the day begin!

It is amazing what effect a day has on your mental state. It's Saturday and the atmosphere at Gabriella's Centre confirmed it. It was so purposefully relaxed. "The nurses at the centre are stunning people, always friendly and loving", I thought to myself. Jamie was fast asleep in his chair. NO wheezing! He seemed very relaxed. I pushed him in his chair to his room and started to prepare. For a moment I thought he peeked through his lovely long eye lashes, but before I could check they fell closed again.

I suspected that this whole week was probably quite intense for him, so I decided to give him a Saturday programme. He was so relaxed I could easily lift up his legs for the cross-crawl. No "will-not-iology" today, just pure relaxation. It was so comforting to see. The nurse told me he had had very few fits this week and when he did they were not very intense. Eureka!
For the next sequence I did two positive tapping sequences, just affirming, what we had been doing during the week. I then rubbed his "energy buttons".

There were no reactions other than his lip curling up. He gave one big snore. "I get the picture Mister Jamie, you are tired," I thought to myself, smiling. I did one more sequence of tapping on "Letting go of the trauma in the cell memories". I stroked his legs very softly and noticed the goose bumps showing up all over. I tested this on his arms and slowly, but surely, the same reaction occurred. I picked him up, gave him a big hug and put him back in his chair. I solemnly wondered if he would know I was here, or would he think I hadn't come.

Let us take the weekend for what it is...The weekend. Let's see what tomorrow and next week will bring. Everything has a time, everything has a purpose and our patience is the vehicle that will determine if we will appreciate the scenery of the journey.

"The mind is a useful servant, but a bad master" –Rebazar Tarz

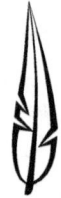

5 BEAUTY LIES IN "MY" EYES

During the past seven days so many things were highlighted about myself, my views of change and the process of development. The protocols and programming of the whole physiological system in individuals have also been reiterated in these sessions. I know procedures can change to facilitate efficiency of functions, but I wrestled with the thoughts on emphasizing emotional change or rather physiological change.

There were so many physiological thing that needed correcting, I felt completely overwhelmed on where to start.
Although there are many different procedures and processes and countless differences in individuals, the process I started to use and feel comfortable with is very simple. Where I like to start, when working with people with disabilities (especially with cerebral palsy), is focusing on the Proprioceptors. Activation or stimulation of proprioceptors will improve communication with the brain.

Proprioceptors are specialized nerve ending that monitor internal changes in the body brought about by movement and muscular activity. They are located in muscles and tendons and transmit information that is used to co-ordinate muscular activity. An easier explanation is that they tell the brain where the body and body parts are.

To help the brain to find the body, you can start at the feet, pulling gently on each joint. This is a time-consuming process and must be done slowly and gently, especially if seizures are present. Until an equilibrium or balance is established, the seizures might increase again. To speed up the process, EFT can be done on proprioceptors which are unable to translate the message received from the brain, the muscles or the tendons.

I have used the following diagram to guide the process of EFT.

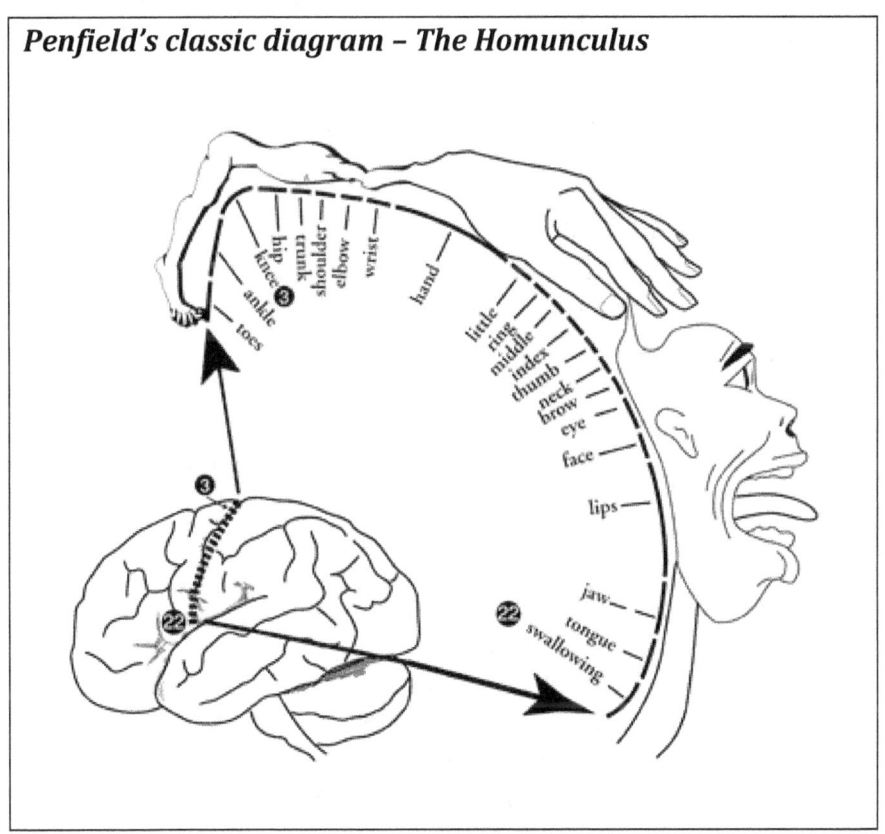

Penfield's classic diagram – The Homunculus

Image can be found on the following website: http://www.intropsych.com/ch02_human_nervous_system/02 homunc.jpg

I usually start at the toes and feet, then go on to the ankles, knees, hip, trunk, shoulder, elbow, wrist, hand, little finger, ring finger, middle finger, index finger and thumb. Then follows the neck, brow, eyelid and eyeball, face, mouth, tongue. Remember to set a clear intention. If this process sounds like a tedious task you can do EFT on general proprioceptors, but I found that using EFT on symptoms and being specific works the best. For example tapping on communication between the brain and the toes. This can be done with all the body parts as stated above. Below is the diagram of the homunculus. I use this diagram to determine the order in which I am going to stimulate the proprioceptor – starting at the toes and working my way up to the neck.

KC: Even though my brain can't find my knees I love and accept myself.
EB: Where are my knees?
SE: I see them but can't feel them.
UE: Maybe I am close to discovering my knees.
UN: Then I can bend them.
CH: New pathways can always be formed.
CB: I can imagine feeling my knees.
UA: But I am still wondering where the feeling is in my knees.
TH: When will the knees and the brain start to communicate?
EB: Are they angry with each other?
SE: Hello, there are my knees.
UE: The brain just needs to see them.
UN: They must really start to communicate.
UM: Brain please see my knees.
CB: Did the communication get lost?
UA: NO, it only has taken another path.
TH: It is in the process of discovering the knees.
Now you might want to ask me "How can you talk to a person if they can't understand you?" Well, firstly, I can honestly say that

the assumption that they can't understand could be wrong. Secondly, I believe all children understand intention of actions and words. Silence your own reservation and work with them as if the sky is your limit.

Another therapist said to me a while ago that I shouldn't give people false hope. My response to her was: "Although in medical cases there aren't many who succeed, as is true in life as well, the bottom line is there ARE some that succeed and there ARE some that improve. Some is better than none. The responsibility that we have is to give the child the opportunity and the benefit of the doubt as if he or she is on their way to recovery. We cannot let our own limiting beliefs inhibit their performance or improvement."

"Why can we do it with children without special needs and tell them the sky is the limit and everything is possible but neglect it when working with children with special needs. Those who persevere are those who leave victoriously.

The other way of using EFT is to focus on the emotional trauma. It can be most beneficial using EFT on not understanding what is happening, or struggling to express or communicate. Sometimes when this emotional trauma is cleared many wonderful things start to happen. When working with people with disabilities it is of the utmost importance to listen to your intuition as well. Sometimes the block or trauma isn't complex at all and it can be cleared in an instant.

Remember the human body is a miracle. Please don't let your judgment or opinion inhibit recovery.

Day 7, January 27, 2013

The alarm clock took its revenge this morning and won the race by a "snoozing" 30 minutes. A vivid memory of the story, the Tortoise and the Hare, got me up quickly (I wouldn't want to be the Hare falling asleep under the tree and missing the race – now would I?).

While driving to Gabriella's Centre I noticed that the huge whale advertisement, which I used as my left- turn landmark, has been removed. "A really big shame, because I like whales" – I thought. I wondered when they had taken it down and why?
As always, the atmosphere at the centre was relaxing and calm.

I am always greeted with smiles and happy faces. This morning, I was greeted by the friendly boy of Day 1. Today, however, he had an elephant and a soft orange blow-up bat. He gave me a hug and then left with the nurse. Jamie was in the changing room. I was so happy to see the bright-brown-open-eyed boy today. The "not-so-intense" day did him well yesterday. Today's easy programme will finish Week 1.

It is so exciting. Next week on Sunday, we will have another week's data and footage to compare. We might be able to see a predicted pattern in his performance or maybe measure biorhythm with activities that were done. While doing my necessary preparations, I was stopped in my tracks by a very interesting and questioning thought. "Who is the teacher and who is the student, Mister Jamie?" Over the past days, I had the wonderful privilege to be taught valuable life lessons by a boy, without him ever saying anything. Wow, that is true and honest magical divinity.

We started the session as we always do. Jamie was wonderfully relaxed and awake and his eyes noticed everything. It seemed as if his muscles were cramping during the massage and stimulation. "Probably, because the "active time" increased," – I thought. During the eighth minute of the session his mouth and arm muscles contracted for about 30 seconds. He followed every movement that I did with his feet, legs, arms and fingers. His eyes were brilliant today, so focused.

We started an EFT tapping sequence on brain communication and pathways. His arms contracted for 15 seconds during the

34th minute of the session, I briefly stopped to check if it was a serious matter. It went as soon as it came and I continued with the tapping. After the sequence his eyes were as bright as ever. I gave him a hug and a kiss and said goodbye.

I have some homework to do before tomorrow. So far we have had five out of seven, in favour of good days. That is a great score! However, there is always room for improvement. May you have a pleasant Sunday Mister Jamie and great excitement for another Monday.

Day 8, January 28, 2013

"No expectations", is the thought that gently walked through my mind and woke me up this morning. Today is a new day and the only expectation I will have is: whatever happens, is the best that will happen today. The thought comforted me quickly and I let go of the control button once again.

"Just have fun", I thought as I quickly jumped up and arranged today's programme. I felt completely grounded in contentment. Today we were going to do a whole new programme, full of fun, colours and a lot of positive tapping. My hand-puppet will be "contracted" to translate for me, to "child-nese".

I arrived very early at the centre this morning because there were a lot of things I had to set up before we could start. The song I got a feeling, from Black Eyed Peas, was stuck in my head as I got out of my car. Mondays, so far, are very good for Jamie (contrary to the general feeling about Mondays). He was wide awake and looked ready for action. Excellent! Today was going to be a great day.

I even got a great big smile this morning when he entered the room. I placed a movement mat on the floor and softly laid him down on it. While I was massaging his feet I gave him a little rubber fish to hold in his hand and to look at. His eyes were amazing, and followed the fish everywhere. I did some sensory integration and his arm shot up. I looked carefully to see if it was a seizure. He glanced at me and I started to tickle his stomach. He suddenly started to laugh. His laugh was genuine and his eyes confirmed it. (Video of laughing can be seen at http://www.youtube.com/watch?v=JVUTbn_Vzm0.) That was my highlight of the session.

We did some more eye-function exercises. I then wanted to start with a tapping sequence, but he was facing the wall. I asked him to turn his head and look at me. I could see how the head was trying to turn. The muscles and brain were communicating. I started with a tapping sequence. Karate chop: "even though not everything is working properly in my body yet, I deeply and completely love and accept myself". Jamie gave a huge yawn and watched every movement intently while I was tapping. I noticed that he looked straight at me every time I spoke to him. We did two more tapping sequences and then did the "Good-bye" song with a hug. Today was truly a good day and I am so grateful.

Day 9, January 29, 2013

A friendly laughing, Jamie, greeted me this morning. He "talked" all the way to his room. A happy, playful sound. What a great start!! The session today, like yesterday, was colourful, bright and full of laughter. After the start-up I did a quick tapping sequence.

He laughed when I picked him up from his chair, when I tickled his cheeks and even when I lifted his shoulders during the massage. We did a lot of singing while doing movements. I made songs up for everything we did. He made many little noises with the songs; it almost seemed as if he was singing along. He smiled when I sang "The Wheels of the Bus" while making rolling movements with his arms. His legs where strong today and I could feel how the muscles were working together with the cross-crawl and leg bending exercises.

Next up for today's fun festival, I switched on a colourful light ball and did some sensory integration. He seemed to be intrigued with the beautiful lights. The light ball swiftly reminded me of the movie, Madagascar 3 (which I'd watched with my two-year-old in the early hours of the morning, twice, because she refused to sleep). I smiled at the colourful and crazy thought. The comparison today was quite appropriate, because Jamie was absolutely amazing.

For last part of the session we did two longer tapping sequences, incorporating and, hopefully, strengthening the ones which we did in the past couple of days. In today's session there where, undoubtedly "no" cramps or fits, just pure joy. With the"Good-bye" song, I got a beautiful smile again from this small angel and, with a big hug; I put him back into his chair. One of the nurses greeted him and spoke to him in a friendly way, when I pushed him into the kitchen and, once again, he laughed.

Happiness filled my whole being, when I left the centre and I fell into an euphoric state. The rationalist in my head, tried to bring me back to earth without success. The reasoning of what tomorrow might or might not bring was completely irrelevant. All that mattered was today. The present moment was truly a great gift. "Thank you, thank you, thank you, Mister Jamie", I thought. "You have finally taught me the significance of appreciating The Now."

For now, I will leave what tomorrow might deliver, in tomorrow's inbox and just enjoy today. I encourage you, the reader, to do the same. Choose the beauty that you would like your eyes to see and then look for it with persistence.

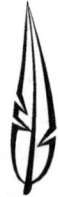

6 OPENING MY HEART TO HEAR THE SOUL

"Divine Grace is not limited by the conditions of ability, but
ability in fact is conditioned by Divine Grace."
-Jalal-ad-Di-ar-Rumi

Every day was an adventure and I was filled with a charge and
a burst of energy which I haven't experienced for a while. I
could feel how my heart was opening up. Suddenly life had
returned and I felt whole, not mended, but whole.

I realised that showing someone unconditional love was an
immense blessing. Not only did I have the opportunity to take a
journey of a lifetime, I, myself, had started to heal.

I remembered reading an article that explained that emotion is
first felt by the heart then by the head. It made perfect sense to
me and I could understand the word "heartfelt" much better.

"Love makes us patient, understanding and kind
And we judge with our heart, not with our mind
For as soon as love enters heart's open door,

The faults we once saw are not there anymore."
– Author unknown

Day 10, January 30, 2013

Day 10 started with a BANG!!! When I got into my car this morning I was overwhelmed by the angelic scent I used in my therapy sessions. This could only mean ONE thing... the bottle was open!!! "GRRRRR!" I growled at myself and then started to laugh.

"Does this mean my car was touched by an angel last night?" Thankfully, it was only the diffusion of the oil through the bottle cap. It reminded me that things (or people) that are so good, can't be contained. Their presence spontaneously just grows bigger than the bottle because the intention is pure enough to make a breakthrough.

When I arrived at the centre the nurse told me Jamie had a stuffy chest and that I needed to do some "pounding on his back" to get it right. I smiled and thought, "Strange how we always think that we can solve everything if we force it?"

"Whatever you resist, persists" - Carl G. Jung. Eckhart Tolle said "Whatever you fight, you strengthen..."

This is why I love using EFT/ Tapping. It never works against something that is, but it channels that something, towards what it can and should become. It isn't forceful, restrictive or even resistant. EFT or tapping is a loving and gentle technique which releases and rekindles energy into something creative and positive.

Qigong expert Chunyi Lin explained in his Spring Forest Healing fest, that energy can't be good or bad, but the application thereof, however, matters.

The nurse lovingly placed Jamie on the mat today and we could start our 10th session. When I had finished with my usual startup, I did a tapping sequence for his lungs and phlegm.

Karate chop and start-up statement: "Even though I have these wheezing lungs today and a lot of phlegm, I deeply and completely love and accept myself."

"Even though I have all this phlegm on my lungs and throat, I deeply and completely love and accept myself."

"Even though I have all this phlegm on my lungs and throat, I deeply and completely love and accept myself."

EB: These lungs of mine.

SE: These wheezing lungs of mine.

UE: All this unnecessary phlegm.

UN: All this phlegm.

CP: All this phlegm

Jamie suddenly started to cough and the phlegm came out. As on Day 4, he stopped wheezing completely and the gurgling noises were gone again. I finished with the tapping sequence all the way to the crown-point on top of the head. Again, this completely amazed me. "Can this be a coincidence that it worked twice in a row?" I asked the critics in my head.

Silencing them quickly, I moved on to the other activities. The toes were very active and moved up and down with each stroke. I did a neck and head massage, while rubbing the ears. I tried to imagine and focus on his neck muscles, visualizing that they were strong.

This was followed by a tapping sequence of the neck muscles. Karate chop and start-up statement: Even though I struggle to keep my neck up, for long periods of time... I deeply and completely love and accept myself. We did two tapping sequences. He gave another big cough and I quickly placed him in recovery position, to get rid of the phlegm.

He was very peaceful and calm and his breathing supported this. I picked him up and held him on my knee, sang the "Good-bye" song, while he looked me squarely in the eyes. What a beautiful sight! I stood up and placed him in his wheelchair. His eyes were wide open and awake. "All is well, everything is going to be okay, and I am safe." With these words of Louise Hay, I pushed him in his wheelchair to the communal room and said good bye.

Day 11, January 31, 2013

"Where are the fires for us to believe in?
Where are the tongues of flames to lick and conquer the dark?
In answer...
The black body of the sky rose up
Loud with the rumbling voices of the stars"

Extract from a poem by Jennifer Davis

Never underestimate the power of one lit candle. It can sow havoc if used for the wrong cause or it can light a million more flames and increase a warm loving light.

Today I could clearly see the stars from the darkness. There was a whole new vibe surrounding Jamie. He didn't smile when I greeted him but his session was purposefully successful. I could feel it every moment he was working with me. He was seemingly listening attentively to every word I was saying, while watching every movement. He seemed very serious today, almost businesslike.

I started with a prayer to open my intuition and our session began. I used a soft blue rubber toothbrush to stimulate the inside of his mouth. When I used the flat end on the other side, he opened and closed his jaws repeatedly almost as if he was chewing. I massaged the mouth and jaw muscles.

The massage and stimulation went very well. I started at his feet and he wiggled the toes on both feet. His right side was a bit more responsive but the left side was still not out of the race. His left ankle seemed stiff and his left foot seemed sore and a bit swollen. I wondered if it was related to his toe that got hurt the other day. I did some gentle massage on the ankle and I told him I was pulling all the hurt out. We moved to both knees. I encouraged him to keep his knees bent and in a static position. This time the left side won by a mile. Massaging of the hands, fingers and shoulders followed.

The noise factors were very disruptive today. Outside I could hear some construction work happening, the garbage truck loading and, every now and again, someone coming into the room. Jamie, however, wasn't fazed by it at all. We continued, doing cycling movements with his legs. We worked together beautifully and we could do 20 sets continuously. We did the same movements on his shoulders, bringing them up and down, alternately. I picked his arm up, holding it in the air, and then encouraged him to keep it there. The left side won again. Stunning! His eyes followed attentively.

The improvement in his eyes was amazing. He was very aware and present.
We then did EFT.

Karate chop: This wonderful body of mine.

EB: Not everything is working as it should yet.

SE: Not everything is communicating as it should yet.

UE: But I am getting there.

UN: Processes have been put into place.

CH: Communication has been set up.

CB: Healthy cell memories are facilitating the process.

UA: Everything is fine.

TH: This wonderful, wonderful body of mine. Everything has a time.

EB: Everything has a place.

SE: I am safe.

UE: All these wonderful processes of mine.

UN: Working lovingly together.

CH: To optimally perform.

CB: All these amazing communication networks.

UA: Working in absolute synergy, to reach optimal potential.

TH: This wonderful, wonderful body of mine, Thank you.

Inhale and exhale.

In the second tapping session we did EFT on the seizures.
All went very well. We sang the "Good-bye" song, and again, with a kiss and a hug, I put him in his wheelchair. While pushing him to the front of the centre, I felt very grateful and calm. The noises dimmed away as I was filled with gratitude and contentment.

Day 12, February 1, 2013

Today is, Thursday, the 1st of February 2013 and Day 12 of "30 days with Jamie". The morning started very quickly.
I stared at my two-year-old, still comfortably sleeping: she'd kept us up most of the night. I smiled and shook my head.

My five-year-old princess was negotiating with her father about something. In the distance, I could hear the CICADAS (or as I know them, the sun-beetles) singing. Today is going to be a great (and very hot) day...

The atmosphere at Gabriella Centre is always loving and kind. I quickly set up the room before I went to fetch Jamie. He was without expression this morning and very quiet. I picked him up from his chair and placed him on the mat. I sprayed the lovely scent and did the starting prayer.

I started with tapping. We did EFT on healing. Afterwards I used the blue rubber toothbrush for stimulation of his mouth. He chewed on it with ease. Although it didn't seem as if he was enjoying it. It made perfect sense..." rubber doesn't taste nice on its own", I thought. "Maybe I must put some agave on for taste, the next time I use this," I thought.

His toes were very responsive to the foot massage and they wiggled constantly. I massaged the ankles, knees, hips, coccyx, fingers, hands, wrist, shoulders, back of the neck and head. We did many cycling movements with his legs. They were relaxed and I could easily bend them. I followed this with alternating movements with the arms. I then took his hands and lifted them in a combing movement over his head. After the 10th movement, he suddenly had a seizure. It lasted 15, painful, seconds. My heart stood still and I stopped breathing. Mental note: We are never doing that again.

He was such a trooper. I massaged his face and rubbed his ears while waiting two minutes, before I started again. I then did a tapping sequence on his seizures and followed that by another tapping sequence which I like to call "The phoenix".

Before our "Good-bye" song, a hug and a kiss, we did another tapping sequence on his lungs again. He honoured me with a faint smile when I left. I fell silent while walking to my car. "It is tapping on Tanya again today. I need to let go of the need to control. What is, is, and what will be, will be." After Day 4 I expected so much. I couldn't understand why these symptoms were recurring. In the evening, when everyone had gone to bed, I got up and went to sit in our lounge. Everything was very quiet.

I started to go through the programme and read over my notes for every day since we had started. I read through his file and studied his history. I then tried to imagine the emotions he might have gone through. I did an EFT session on myself, tapping on letting go the need to control. After prayer, I returned to bed and awaited the morning with a breath of fresh air inhaled into my soul.

"All is well, everything is going to be okay and I am safe" – Louise Hay

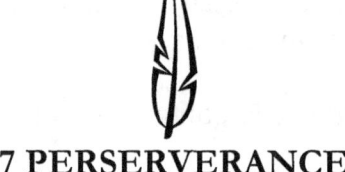

7 PERSERVERANCE

Day 13, February 2, 2013

I was woken up by our cat, Chloe, who was trying to balance on me while I was sleeping on my side. My alarm didn't go off (probably because I forgot to set it) and the house was quiet. Not even the sun- beetles (Cicadas) were singing today. I felt tired. Yesterday was very emotional. I felt like a child hoping my mother or father would jump in and make everything better. I put on my big-girl shoes and, with much bravery, decided to face Day 13.

"What does it mean to trust?
It means to have such inner knowing
That your thoughts create your world,
To simply be quiet certain,
With divine nonchalance and inner knowing,
That if you think something, it is."
From "Bringers of the Dawn" by Barbara Marciniak

The streets were deserted, not even pedestrians were in sight. Only the "Beggar-Budgies" (sparrows) were on the pavements pecking at the memories of yesterday. The gate of the centre opened and it sounded as if the bell was echoing into the fresh morning air. Everything was quite. It seemed like the "Saturday Vibe" was universal and everyone felt it.

Jamie was up and ready, even though yesterday had brought the "good days vs. bad days"- score to 9:3, it was still a great score, I thought. We were told that we could use the communal room today. "Brilliant, a change of scenery would do us good, Mister Jamie," I said jokingly to him.

We started as we always do and quickly moved on to the next few activities. I changed the order of the activities today. First, massage and stimulation of proprioceptors of both feet, both ankles, both knees, the hips and the coccyx. Then we did cycling movements, alternating both legs. I followed that with cross crawl. Before I started with the arms, I did another tapping sequence.

Karate Chop: This body of mine is forming new and healthy cells daily.

The same sequence was followed with fingers, arms, elbows, shoulders and neck, as I had done with the legs. Up and down movements with arms and shoulders followed and lastly the cross-crawl.

This morning we did three tapping sequences. I then rolled him on to his side and pressed next to his spine and his coccyx and gently rubbed his back. When I spoke to him, his neck turned and his eyes looked at me. I was very impressed with his response.

I stood up to get the golden stickers I sometimes stick on his hands. I stuck one on his left hand and then taking a chance I said: "Lift up your hand Jamie." The left hand went up. "Well done! It is now the turn of the other hand."

His right arm was stretched out horizontal to the floor. I realised he was going to need a lot more strength to bring his arm up from that position, than he would have if the arm had been closer to the body. I placed his arm next to his side. Then saying: "Let's start again .... Try lifting your arm, Jamie. I will wait for you. Lift your arm." With a sudden jerking movement he lifted up his arm. I had to check if it wasn't another seizure, but with the smile on his face and his eyes, I knew it wasn't.

He had communicated to his body. The signal took a bit longer, but nonetheless, there was communication and, more importantly, comprehension. Yay, Yay, Yay!! I could see the sense of achievement in his eyes and smile. Stunning. What a way to start the day! Thank you Mister Jamie. The memory of yesterday was wiped out completely. The video can be seen at http://www.youtube.com/watch?v=F-KLRxw_YTk.

"An arrow can be sent forward only by pulling it back. So when life is pulling you backwards, it means it is going to launch you to a victory." Author Unknown

Day 14, February 3, 2013

The Impossible Dream (lyrics written by Joe Darion and composed by Mitch Leigh rang in my ears this morning when I woke up. This is so true, for the little man I will be seeing in an hour.

To have so much courage and determination and not give up the fight even when he was faced by death. Dear brave Jamie. I received a big smile this morning, when I said hello. The victory of yesterday still echoed in our hearts. We started the session in our usual fashion and then moved to sequence two, in the same order as we had done yesterday.

I wanted to try something new. We established yesterday that there was some sort of comprehension. Today I was going to establish if we could get a solid "yes" when I asked a question. "If the answer is yes, please lift your hand," I asked him. "Must we do the cycling again? Lift your arm if the answer is yes."

Every single time he lifted his arm. The last time I asked, he actually didn't lift his arm and I thought I will test it... I started with the cycling movement and suddenly he kicked both legs straight. I smiled and apologised for not recognising his "no". He smiled and looked me in the eyes. I knew we might have a "yes" for now.

I needed to find a way to establish "no" as an answer. I have noticed that sometimes when I asked a question he would roll his eyes upwards. This is still something to be clarified and we will test it, starting tomorrow. He made happy noises while I was singing the songs, almost as if he was singing with me (or maybe urging me to be quiet). If the last were true, he would learn to say "no" very quickly. I gave him a little rubber orange fish as reward and he clenched it in his left hand.

We did two tapping sequences;
1) Body making healthy cells; 2) Everything that happens is for the greater good of him. I then rolled him unto his side and rubbed his back, coccyx and neck.

When I turned him back he suddenly had a seizure, his eyes went wild, going left and right frantically, he clenched his jaw and I could hear the grinding of his teeth. His eyes started to water and he made crying sounds underneath his shallow breathing. The orange fish fell to the floor. The seizure lasted 10 seconds. I held him tight and kissed his cheek.

"Everything that happens is for the greater good of him." I reminded myself. This is easier to believe when there is a victory, rather than when you are still in the battle.
I whispered in his ear; "Everything that happens is for the greater good of you, Mister Jamie. We must believe that with our whole heart. All is well, everything is going to be okay, and you are safe."

Jamie was exhausted when I placed him back into his chair. I pushed him to the communal room; the silence was audible and uncomfortable. I gave him two golden stickers on his hands and said "One day at a time." The boy with the lion from Day 1, snuggled up and gave me a huge hug, almost as if he knew I needed it. I stuck a golden star on his forehead and said he must have a lovely day too...

I left and the silence followed me into my car and into my heart. I suddenly heard myself saying out load "Everything happens to the greater good, you must believe it." – And I do. Nothing and no one can be allowed to steal one's truth...
"We will try again tomorrow Mister Jamie. The "59 minutes and 50 seconds went very well, indeed."

Day 15, February 4, 2013

In the past 15 days, immense improvements have occurred. We have established a way to say "yes". Jamie can comprehend and act on various instructions like: lift up your hand, look at me, look at my finger, wiggle your toes, etc. Today I asked him to open his mouth and stick out his tongue. I could literally see all the planning that was taking place, leading to him widening his mouth and sticking out his tongue a little bit. It seemed as if there was a swallowing reflex, because it seemed as if he was swallowing his saliva. This needed to be confirmed.

With a lot of planning and patience, he could lift various parts of his body and when he felt he has had enough exercise he would straighten his legs or pull back his arm. His eyes were much more coordinated. He acted on sounds and had become a lot more vocal.

There was one big reservation; however. The frequency of his seizures was increasing. He had four seizures in the past five days, while in session. This was somewhat worrisome. I had a slight suspicion that his medicine needed to be adjusted. I decided to address this theory in the next few days. The whole idea of different therapies and therapists was that the one must compliment, strengthen and facilitate the other. "Synergy" is a word that I like to use a lot...

I was a little disappointed that a few symptoms kept on returning and I thought the retention of improvements wasn't very good. A few days ago, I started to study his background and write down all the possible emotions he might have gone through and all the possible traumatic events. I read through Louise Hay's book, You can heal your life, countless times, as possible reference, to emotions that could possibly cause illness.

I have imagined myself in his situation so many times. This immense fever, people panicking, the pain that didn't stop. Possible negative things people said and then waking up, all alone in a strange place. He probably felt forgotten, overlooked, disconnected, lonely and angry. I started to incorporate all of these traumatic events and emotions into our sessions.

Some might say ALL disorders or illnesses are linked to emotions. I say we are holistic human beings with many influences in our lives. There must be some room left for the possibility that healing and illnesses are an integrated process. If a child is born normal with no defect or disability there still lays a responsibility and task to keep his milestones on track, either by his parents, teacher or therapist. First we learn to move then we learn through movement. It is a process, a much-needed process.

Jamie was in such a good mood today, very vocal. His "consciously aware" time was increasing daily. His sessions were now an hour long and most of the time he was "there", watching and responding. His arms were lifting up and down. The right arm responded with more difficulty. For our halfway mark session, we sang a few "move-together" songs. He smiled each time I asked him "Must we do it again? Lift your arm if you say yes or look up if the answer is no," and he would lift his arm. Each time I wanted to start the tapping sequence he would pull his hand away and smile. It is good to see the playful Jamie. I tapped on his hand and not on his face today.
I told him a story about an ant and an elephant and then I

showed him a story of the ant and the grasshopper (on my Samsung tablet), where he had to use his pointing-finger to feed the grasshopper. I rolled him on to his back again and suddenly he rolled back on his side. (I am still not sure how he did that.)

We started with the arms and suddenly he cringed with pain (another seizure), and it left him weeping on the floor. Then it was over and it almost seemed as if it never happened. The seizures, in our session, were violently worse these last couple of days. I did a last tapping sequence – no words, just tapping, the body would know what he needed now.

He was completely relaxed when I pushed him to the kitchen, where they were getting ready for breakfast. See you tomorrow Mister Jamie, the second half is usually the determining factor... "No pressure, Tanya, no pressure!!!"

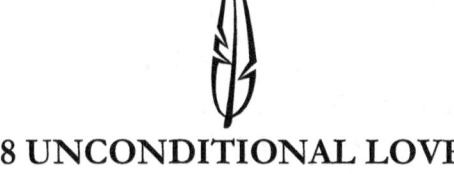

8 UNCONDITIONAL LOVE

Day 16, February 5, 2013

Day 16, the first day of the second half...

I was nervous as I entered the centre and my mouth felt dry, as it did in the first week. Although the excitement and curiosity still had the upper hand there was still so much we needed to do and time was waiting for no one.

Jamie was fast asleep when the nurse pushed him into the room. I kissed him on the cheek and his mouth lifted as if he was smiling. I kissed him on the other cheek and he opened his eyes and I could clearly see he was smiling. I lifted him from his chair and placed him on the movement mat.

"Look at the beautiful legs," I said and it seemed as if he was trying to lift or move them. I said it again and he did it again. It seemed as if he had a little bit of an infection because thick white phlegm was visible in his mouth. I could see the permanent teeth making their appearance behind his baby teeth. He is growing into a big boy now.

The nurse quickly came to change him and used glycerine sticks to clean his mouth. With everything happening, he actually didn't seem sick. He gave a big cough and I jokingly said: "This naughty phlegm, I think I must catch it and smack its bum." He smiled as if he knew I was making a joke (or maybe thinking "this lady is crazy, just smile and maybe she will go away".)

After commencing the session as I usually do, I immediately continued with a tapping sequence on the fear of life. I then, rubbed his back, neck and coccyx, I swiftly moved to his feet. "Wiggle your toes Jamie," I said. "Come on wiggle your toes." He did just that.

Stunning! A nurse came in to get something and I thought I would try it again. "Wiggle your toes Jamie, come on wiggle your toes." He did it again. The nurse smiled in amazement and we both praised him. I then started with the foot and leg massage.

Another tapping sequence followed. We tapped on the medicine he was using and that everything had a positive effect and that nothing had any negative effects. With all the activities our time was up very quickly. I did one more tapping sequence on feeling overlooked and picked him up and placed him in the chair.

"I am excited to see how you will astonish us Mister Jamie. You have come so far in 15 days; imagine what might happen in the next... " I stopped myself in my own tracks. Improvements can't be forced or measured in time. Everything has its own time and place.

"My prayer for you is, Mister Jamie, that now will be your time to shine and that your potential will outstretch and out climb your circumstances and history and that we acknowledge that every day is a victory. Amen."

Day 17, February 6, 2013

"If you always put a limit on everything you do, physical or anything else. It will spread into your work and into your life. There are no limits. There are only plateaus, and you must not stay there, you must go beyond them."

- Bruce Lee

While listening to Nick Ortner last night (The Tapping World Summit 2013) my wonderful husband and I came to a life-changing realisation. We realised that our (the human race's) reservations usually create our own limitations. For instance: Before we can be healthy we must first join a gym, before we can start a business we must first have a lot of money or I can only be healthy once I have started to eat healthily. The above-mentioned reasons are so limiting and are only the tip of the iceberg.

The desire to change, must be much greater than your need to stay the same" so, if you want to live healthily it can only start by a decision that, from today I am healthy and I will listen to what my body needs. It can be possible to start a business by putting up one poster at a supermarket or advertising on all the free business advertising sites.

We subconsciously like to stay in our comfort zone (even when it isn't comfortable at all). We'd rather complain and blame than get up and start doing something about it. You always have something to give (so that you can receive), whether it is time, effort, love or even a smile to brighten someone's day.

With this mind set, I drove peacefully to Gabriella Centre this morning. "The body knows what the body needs, we can only facilitate the process and the intention has already been set". This thought released my control button completely as well as all my limiting beliefs and reservations.

We started with the session very quickly, Jamie was awake and ready. I have noticed his state of alertness works in three phases. If he is awake it takes five to ten minutes to become aware when we start the session, then approximately another ten minutes to successfully start to interact and then the last phase is to spontaneously move and "communicate". The three phases have moved closer every day and his "aware" time has increased dramatically.

We started the session and swiftly moved to the next activities. His muscles were very relaxed. He wiggled his toes, assisted with the ankle rotations and leg bends. I have noticed that I don't have to press the "leg buttons" anymore for him to bend his legs. I need only touch the back of the leg and it will relax.

We moved to the hands and he lifted his left hand when I asked him to. The right arm was still a little stubborn and the reaction time was very slow, but I was very grateful that there was a reaction. I could see the muscles trying to contract and then, after a long wait, the arm shot up again. The smile on his face and the sense of achievement was priceless. I turned him on his side and worked on his back, coccyx and neck. There was no thick white phlegm today and I was so grateful.

I did some tapping on his hands and feet. He watched carefully. Then I did this EFT sequence. To me, it felt powerful and so on par.

EFT on healing the body

Karate chop -The body knows what the body needs and what it wants, the body knows what it can use and what it can't. The body knows.

EB - the body knows how to heal itself; the body knows how to make new cells.

SE: The body knows how to make new healthy cells. How to get rid of old unhealthy cells.

UE: The body knows how to make new motor pathways and how to prepare the brain.

UN: This wonderful body of mine that knows how to prepare itself, how to repair itself.

CH: This wonderful body of mine, repairing itself daily, forming new cells.

CB: Using cell memories of generations, using good cell memories of generations.

UA: This body of mine, this body of mine knows no time, it only knows now.

TH: This body of mine is not shackled to time limits, is not influenced by negative views.

EB: This body of mine knows no limits; this body of mine is open to miracles.

SE: And allows healing.

UE: This body of mine is open to that wondrous power of healing and enlightenment.

UN: That wondrous power which we call the Light and Love.

CH: This body of mine is open to heal.

CB: This wonderful body of mine is open to wondrous miracles to occur in my life.

UA: This wonderful body of mine is preparing itself daily.

TH: This body of mine is making new cells, thousands, millions, trillions of them and it facilitates this healing process.

EB: This wonderful body of mine, I love life, life loves me.

SE: I take in each breath with gratitude each sight with gratitude, every smell with gratitude, every taste, every sound every feeling, every circumstance.

UE: I take life in with gratitude and I open myself to the endless possibilities in me, I open myself to the endless wondrous possibilities in me.

UN: Everything is going to be ok. All is well, I am safe.

CH : The light above me, the light to the left of me, light to the right of me, light in front of me, light at the back of me, light underneath me, lights everywhere.

CB: I love life, life loves me.

UA: I am open and receptive to receive all the wonderful gifts that God has in store for me.

TH: I am open and receptive for the good in life.

This EFT came so naturally. I wasn't sure if it was intended for him or for me.

For the last EFT sequence we did the following tapping sequence, which I have found to be very helpful when tapping on health issues and you are not quite sure where to start. Anyone can use it. Thinking about your health issues, on a scale from 1 to 10, (1 being very good and 10 being very bad), where are you at? Say the problem out load, for instance: "I am not very healthy." Write down your score.

Karate chop: Even though I don't feel very healthy because..., I am in the process of sorting my health out.

EB: I don't feel very healthy.

SE: I actually feel very sick, especially in my.

UE: I have tried everything or I don't know where to start.

UN: I really feel sick.

CH: How am I going to sort it out?

CB: I don't want to take forever sorting this out.

UA: I want to sort it out now.

TH: Maybe I must open myself up to heal.

EB: Maybe I can imagine myself as being healthy.

SE: No, I can't.

UE: I am not healthy.

UN: I am actually in a very poor shape.

CH: Maybe I am exaggerating.

CB: Maybe I can consider that my body is busy healing.

UA: Maybe I can consider that my body knows what I need.

TH: Everything has a process.

Day 18 – February 7, 2013.

"The power of God gives only what we take."- Anonymous

Case study 4

A woman, who I will call Jane, came to see me. She was very religious. A few things in her life struggled to fall into place, her love life and finances were among them. Judging on face value she seemed happy and enlightened.

After a few EFT sequences and a little digging, we came to the realisation that she didn't believe that she deserved to be blessed and that she wasn't worthy. All the gratitude and belief that she showed to others was not true in her own life, because of this limiting belief.

We did EFT on not feeling worthy or deserving to be blessed. It became apparent to me that sometimes we asked and prayed for something but didn't believe we should receive it.

A loud and very hollow "THUMP" echoed into the early hours of the morning... I opened my eyes and my husband was looking at me, puzzled. "What are you doing?" he asked. I could see he wanted to burst into laughter, but instead he tried to look worried or concerned. I was still too confused to get the joke. I heard my little girl moaning in her room and, with my very numb legs; I tried to walk to her room. I picked her up and put her in our bed. We said nothing...

Later that morning we had a chance to discuss the "early- in- the- morning- event"... I had been fast asleep and in the distance I could hear my little girl crying. I got such a fright that I wanted to jump up and run to her.

Unfortunately there were a delay in communication to my legs and as soon as I got up I realised that I had no legs to stand on, thus falling on to my dresser and bouncing on to the bed and then falling on to the floor. I must have looked like a rubber bouncing-ball or like a pinball machine.

Even now I can't stop laughing when I think of that evening. If there had been a camera in our room when it happened, I would surely have won something. The puzzled expression on my husband's face and then me walking like Igor (from the movie Frankenstein) to my little one's room, because at night when she calls for mommy" SHE ONLY WANTS MOMMY !!!", was absolutely hilarious. I decided that serious Tapping must be done on my body's communication network...

The road was very busy today and everyone seemed to be in a hurry. I wondered if I had missed a memo of some sort. The friendly nurses at Gabriella Centre told me Jamie was still sleeping. They were busy changing Jamie's nappy in the changing room.

I quickly set up the room and the camera. He was fast asleep when the nurse brought him in. I kissed his cheeks and there were no response. I slowly picked him up and carefully placed him on the movement mat. His breathing was slow, deep and relaxed. Today we would be doing more or less the same programme as on Day 6, I have decided. Very relaxed.

The massage was soft and relaxing, so was the stimulation of the joints. I used the tapping point on the feet and the hands and just ran through a few tapping sequences, no words just tapping. The body knows. I then moved to the same tapping sequence I did yesterday. He was very relaxed.

After 45 minutes I picked him up and placed him back into his chair. His eyes opened, although he still seemed to be asleep. I pushed him to the kitchen. "Please tell him I was here, just in case he doesn't remember" I told the nurse. "You must have a great day Mister Jamie. Rest and I will see you tomorrow."

When I left I said to one of the nurses "This was an amazing session". She replied:"God is good". No, God is great, I thought while smiling. I am so happy and grateful. Thank you, thank you, and thank you!

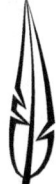

9   A PRISONER OF MY THOUGHTS

"A mind enclosed in language is in prison."
- Simone Weil

In the past few days, the blog, which I was writing about this journey, became very popular and viewings shot up. People all over the world were sending love and well wishes to Jamie. I sat back in my chair and stared in amazement. For so long, I have been locked up in my own head and focusing on my losses and failures. Ironically, I was the one who used to feel completely trapped. After starting this case study, something began to shift. I felt alive, happy and free. Here was this angel of a boy who was not able to leave his room on his own, nor say a word and yet he was able to reach thousands of people all over the world.

"For it was not into my ear, you whispered but into my heart. It was not my lips you kissed but my soul." – Judy Garland

The importance of the power of thought echoed in my head. We hear it a lot and often refer to it but some of us very seldom apply it. I was reading an article and the following emphasised the importance of thought:

In a fascinating experiment, researchers at the Cleveland Clinic Foundation discovered that a muscle can be strengthened just by thinking about exercising it.

For 12 weeks (five minutes a day, five days per week) two teams of 30 healthy young adults imagined either using the muscles of their little finger or of their elbow flexor. Dr Vinoth Ranganathan and his team asked the participants to think as strongly as they could about moving the muscles being tested, to make the imaginary movement as real as they could. Compared to a control group – which did no imaginary exercises and showed no strength gains – the little-finger group increased their pinkie muscle strength by 35%. The other group increased elbow strength by 13.4%. (Neuropsychologia 42 (2004) 944–956)

Day 19 – February 8, 2013

Last night the weirdest and the most wonderful thing happened. I received an email stating that something I really wanted to do was already paid for. I was in absolute AWE. It placed me in a whole different mind-set... one of "anything is possible"... We always say it, but we don't really always feel it.

I was so ready, when I arrived at Gabriella Centre. The "everything is possible" –headset was now on and I felt it pumping through my veins. What an amazing feeling...

Jamie was sleeping peacefully and I instinctively knew his body was working hard to repair and restore itself. I started with the session. I could see his eyes moving rapidly underneath his eyelids almost like a REM phase. I wondered if he was dreaming and, if he was, what was he dreaming about?

His breathing was slow and relaxed and there was no phlegm. I did EFT on "this amazing body and that the body knows what it needs". It lasted eight minutes. He woke up 30 minutes after the session started. I worked on his face muscles. He kept on stretching and yawning. Every now and again I saw a glimpse of a smile. I kept on asking him to say hello, I could see his mouth trying to move and I kept on nagging and nagging and nagging. This "everything is possible" feeling was just not satisfied yet.

I could hear different throat noises... After one minute he gave a response... On the video you could see my face and delayed reaction. I first sat there open mouthed then my reaction came.

That was amazing. A glimpse of a smile was all over his face. He actually looked a little mischievous. He suddenly seemed so awake, almost as if he was looking for something. I calmed his breathing and we did one last tapping sequence of feeling disconnected and the being rejected.

I picked him up, kissed his cheeks, sang the "Good-bye" song and placed him back into his chair.

When I got back to the office I received another e-mail stating that yesterday's email was sent in error. I intuitively knew it wasn't an error. It was a very important lesson to learn – if I am expecting miracles I must be feeling it as well, then miracles can start to happen. That dear "anything great can happen" – feeling.

Thank you e-mail I received in error, you have made my day!!! Dear reader, have a happy "anything great can happen" day!

Day 20- February 9, 2013

Soft rain has been falling since early this morning. Soft rain has a special connotation for me. It reminds me of God's Grace and I feel blessed.

Everyone was still sleeping when I left this morning. In a way, I felt alone and the empty streets emphasised this feeling. It was Saturday and was Day 20. I can't believe how quickly time has flown by. Jamie's mum has informed me that together with the paediatrician, they have decided to decrease the dosage of one of his medicines. We will be monitoring him closely for the next few days. He has been taking this medicine from the beginning.

I have done a tapping sequence on this and I will continue for the rest of the sessions to make sure the body will adapt. This is, however, a learning curve for all of us and I am so grateful that his parents are willing and supportive.

As always, the relaxing Saturday feeling was blooming at the centre. The atmosphere at the centre was serene and clean but not at all like a hospital. It has a very homely feel, full of love. The nurse brought Jamie to the room. Today he was awake. The sleeping marathon he had done the past two days had done him a lot of good.

I picked him up and placed him on the mat. His muscles felt stiff today, especially his right leg and hands. When I started with his left foot, he started to cough and he turned himself on his side. I placed him in recovery position and quickly changed the order of the activities, to work on his back, neck and coccyx. When I turned him on his back again, he had a seizure which lasted less than 20 seconds. His eyes rolled up and he clenched his fists with all his might, his legs curled in. I stroked his arms and back while he was lying in the foetal position. There were no tears and no teeth grinding.

I changed my focus completely and started a tapping sequence. Karate chop – "Even though this brain of mine caused this whole situation, I deeply and completely love and accept myself. Even though this brain of mine, with it self-destructive programming, is keeping me here I deeply and completely love and accept myself." Even though this brain of mine caused everything, I deeply and completely love and accept myself."

I suddenly felt angry...

EB: I am very angry with the brain.

SE: Very angry with my brain.

UE: How must it correct itself with this programming?

UN: This brain of mine, trapping me.

CH: "With its self-destruct button.

CB: Why?

TH: Why do I have this, why are you trapping me?

EB: I was so young.

SE: The brain that is supposed to help me.

UE: Is trapping me.

Frustration was building up...

UN: I want to scream in frustration.

CH: Arrrrrrrrgh.

CB: I am so frustrated.

UA: I am very, very frustrated and angry.

TH: I am so angry.

I kept on tapping until I felt the intensity of the feeling was going down. It was a very emotional EFT sequence for me. Jamie repeatedly yawned throughout the sequence. I moved to the next activities on practising "hello," lifting hands, arms and wiggling toes.

Then I did EFT on letting the negative programming go. Afterwards we sang "the Wheels on the Bus" and "Let's Bake Cake" while making movements with the songs. Lastly, I sang the "Good-bye" song and, with a kiss and a hug, I placed him back into his chair. "All is well, everything is okay, and I am safe." I told him and myself. A 55 minutes session. "Well done."

I have asked the nurses to repeat and strengthen certain stimuli like: "Say hello Jamie", "Lift your arm Jamie" and any other basic instructions, after I have left. His comprehension is good; we must use it to his advantage. The rain continued to fall and I felt truly grateful...

Day 21 – February 10, 2013

The cat's fight club was held outside our bedroom window last night, and there were a few rematches during the course of the night and into the early hours of the morning. Through the commotion, my thoughts travelled to Taylor Jill Bolte, writer of the book: My Stroke of Insight: A Brain Scientist's Personal Journey. This book describes her eight- year journey to recovery after she had a stroke that damaged the left hemisphere of her brain.

Although Taylor, herself, had to work hard together with different therapists, most of her motivation and help came from those truly seeing that she was still there on the inside. Truly seeing her potential even though all the facts and evidence were against her. They were willing to work with what she had and slowly and surely kept on raising the bar.

There is an online video of the author dramatically discussing what her journey:
http://www.ted.com/talks/jill_bolte_taylor_s_powerful_stroke _of_insight.html

My thoughts immediately searched through memories and files of yesterday and possibilities of tomorrow that have been stored or maybe trashed. How many possibilities and wonders have we been neglected and how many limiting beliefs have we been entertaining and strengthening? How short-sighted we are as humans. The phrase "seeing, is believing" should be a perfect example of this HUGE limiting belief...We will start to believe in wonder when wonder shows up on our front porch with flowers and a tuxedo. Tisk-tisk. All these terms and conditions.

Jamie was right and ready, waiting for me in the communal room. His breathing was slow and relaxed and his eyes were wide open. Stunning! I pushed him in his wheelchair to the room. I picked him up, kissed his soft cheeks and placed him on the mat. His eyes watched me carefully while starting the session and, as soon as I started to massage the feet, he began to cough and again turned himself on his side. I immediately started to work on his back.

The breathing returned to normal and again, he inhaled when I asked him to. I moved to the hands, massaging and stimulating all the bendable parts while naming each part individually. I did an EFT sequence on the hands and fingers that were so tight. I personally believe for one to receive, one's hands must always be open and giving; therefore it was important to me that his hands were open and relaxed.

His fingers relaxed and his hands lay open next to his side. I moved back to the feet, ankles, knees, hips and coccyx. I then started with the cross-crawl. All his muscles felt strong and his arms helped me a little. We practised indicating "hello", and lifting his arm and wiggling his toes. We then did another EFT sequence on feeling forgotten and sang two songs and 60 minutes were over. I picked him up, sang the "Good-bye" song and placed him in his chair. NO SEIZURES TODAY YEAH!!!!!

He was very responsive today and awake and making a lot of throat noises. "Keep it up Mister Jamie! We will take this, one victory at a time, your time." Xxx

The boy with the lion, from Day 1 escorted me out of the gate and with a huge hug he said goodbye. What a privilege!

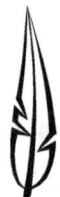

10 ACCEPTING RATHER THAN EXPECTING

To accept a situation for what it is, you give peace permission to take your hand and intuition permission to open your eyes and see how beautiful this situation may become.

Day 22 – February 11, 2013

I found myself procrastinating today and was very reluctant to start typing... I knew what the problem was. After submitting today's blog I only have eight days left and I am definitely not in a hurry to finish them.

The past 22 days have been a very steep learning curve for me, my family and, hopefully, many other people. I have learned that looks can definitely be deceiving and that a true and honest smile can speak a million words if you are willing to listen. I have seen how immense pain can be the only evidence that you are still alive and also how it can make you feel as if you are numb and lifeless on the inside.

I have felt how love for someone else can unlock your own

bleeding heart and free so many locked-up emotions. I have smelled the renewing sweet smells of the outside and started to appreciate each and every breath I have inhaled without a struggle.

The pure bliss of just being able to do things without even thinking about it. I have walked, once again, in the garden of hopes and dreams and realised that some are just an arm's length away while others needed to be revisited and the lessons needed to be learned. I have come to realise that if you make someone believe that they have limitless potential, they can astonish you and themselves.

"What happens when people open their hearts?"...

"They get better." — Haruki Murakami

The awake and aware little boy was pushed into the room. His eyes looked down. "Hello Mister Jamie! What have you been up to while I was away?" I asked. His eyes slanted upward, almost as if he was trying to remember (I knew he was trying to focus and look at me).

I picked him up and hugged and kissed him. Slowly I placed him on the mat. He was now alert and super awake, almost as if he knew that the work was about to start. I did our starting prayer and afterwards said: "Let the games begin." I immediately started with an EFT sequence on strengthening the neck muscles to support the head and assist with breathing.

I then started with the left hand, wrist, elbow, shoulders and neck. Today he kept on pulling back his hand and then smiled at me. When I started with the right wrist he had a HUGE seizure that lasted 30 seconds. It was a really big one. His face turned scarlet and it seemed as if his eyes were bulging out. He made small moaning noises as I held him tightly and kissed his cheek. It took another 30 seconds to return to awareness and relax. Then suddenly it seemed as if the seizure placed him in a higher state of awareness. He was now wide awake and smiling. I wondered if it had something to do with the immense pain stimuli that would secrete a high amount of endorphins that could bring on such a euphoric feeling. I refer to the Endorphin-Rush.

Endorphins function as neurotransmitters and are produced by the pituitary gland and hypothalamus during pain stimuli, exercise and excitement, to name a few. They are very similar to opiates in their ability to produce analgesia and a feeling of well-being. The term "endorphin rush" refers to feelings of exhilaration brought on by the above-mentioned activities or feelings, supposedly due to the influence of endorphins.

Could this possibly mean that there were some working parts in Jamie's hypothalamus and that some sort of regeneration had already started to happen? Maybe there were other working parts but, because of little stimulation or trauma and swelling to the brain, they couldn't be identified? I left my hypothesis right at the exit door and kept on working.

I can't lose focus on the "now". Jamie was a very happy boy for the rest of the session, and laughed when he got something right or when I spoke to him. We did another tapping sequence on this wonderful brain and smooth communication between receptors and that the overwhelming amount of stimuli must be broken down and spread evenly. (Would this work? Honestly, I don't know yet, but the body knows and it will do what is best for him.)

What is important is that the right intention has been set. For the next phase I worked on his feet, ankles, knees, hips and coccyx. He kept on pulling his leg back when I massaged his feet, then he would smile mischievously. He giggled when I massaged his knees. Today his legs felt strong. After one last tapping sequence I picked him up, sang the "Good-bye" song and placed him back in his chair.

He was in a very good mood and laughed when I pushed him in to the communal room. Although I felt bad about him having a seizure, I honestly felt that we had a very good session.

Day 22 was a bitter-sweet-sweet session and I am excited to see what possibilities lay ahead.

Dear Reader, for this day, may you laugh constantly, dance frequently, feel grateful often and every time you can open the door to go outside (whether it is snowing, raining or the sun is blazing), give a thought to all of those (young and old) who can't, and bless them with Love!

Love and Light. Amen

Day 23 – February 12, 2013

"Every cell within our body responds to every single thought you think and word you speak" Louise L. Hay - You Can Heal your Life.

Jamie smiled from ear to ear when I arrived this morning and this carried on throughout the session. He was very happy today and he seemed very playful. He laughed when I spoke to him, tickled him and kissed him on his cheeks. He was very loveable.

After commencing the session, I continued with a sequence on the Corpus Callosum, to support and facilitate communication between the two hemispheres. I then started with the hands, wrists, elbows and shoulders of both his sides. He had a quick eight-second seizure, but was completely aware afterwards. No recovery time was needed or tiredness was present.

I did a tapping sequence on the six triangles of the neck. Then I started with the feet, knees, hips and coccyx. Again his legs felt strong. He started to cough and I turned him on his side to work on the back. The last tapping sequence I did was for the cerebellum. The functions of the cerebellum are to sustain balance, co-ordinate motor activities and regulate the muscle tone. This seemed to be a very important tapping sequence.

Jamie's awareness has increased drastically and because he has become more aware of sensory stimuli, this might make him more susceptible to having more seizers more often (because of sensory overload or inability to process the information). This is why I have decided to scale down on sensory integration activities (for now) and increase the waiting time between tapping sequences. We now do one tapping sequence at the beginning of the session, one in the middle and one at the end. When he became restless, I would tap on his hands and feet rather than on his face.

I watched the videos of the past few days over and over again, studying each expression, reaction and change that occurred. It is apparent, Mister Jamie, there are drastic changes noticeable from Day One to where we are now.

Although some changes happen more slowly in some areas than in others, change is inevitable and the only constant factor. The lesson of change, however, is directly influenced by our ability to adapt. I used to think (when I was very young) it was directly related to our intelligence, but now I know our attitude towards change is the key.

Do we perceive it as an adventurous journey waiting to be explored or an irritating delay that will stay forever because we don't embrace it? Remember what we resist will persist.

I sang the "Good-bye" song, gave him a hug and a kiss and placed him in his chair. "See you tomorrow Mister Jamie".

"The primary cause of unhappiness is never the situation but your thoughts about it."

— Eckhart Tolle, A New Earth: Awakening to our Life's Purpose

Day 24 – February 13, 2013

"Everybody is a genius. But if you judge a fish by its ability to climb a tree, it will live its whole life believing that it is stupid." –

The source of this quote is still highly disputed. None the less, this quote is still very wise and wonderful.

Today started a little bit slower than usual. My head felt like heavy iron and the bed and pillow like a magnet. I could not lift my head to start the process of getting up. This gave me a very good idea what it must feel like to Jamie not being able, yet, to lift his head. And the earth's gravity doesn't make it any easier. I am grateful though that he can breathe more easily now, even when his head is hanging low.

There are so many improvements that we have noted over the past 24 days. His state of awareness has improved drastically, so has his responsiveness. His breathing, phlegm and lungs have improved. I have noticed a lot of heartburn and have advised his parents to start with probiotics again. This will help to adjust the pH to improve the alkalinity. I have noticed in the past three days that his involuntary muscle movement has increased dramatically. The reason for this is not yet 100% clear to me, so it is something to keep an eye on. His seizures have also increased drastically according to the nurses at the centre. We are aware that his body has been used to the medicine from the start of his condition, so the reduction in dosage, definitely plays a role. We must just determine if the body will be able to adapt successfully to the changes and if the seizures lessen?

Time is the only factor which will bring clarity on the matter and, as you all know, time doesn't always come with an appointment. Today's session was very playful. Jamie laughed from the beginning to the end. He kept on pulling his hands away when I started the massage. I did one tapping session on his feet, the other on his hands and the last sequence on the face. We played peek-a-boo and he laughed with great joy.

I turned him on his side to massage his back, neck and coccyx. We went through all the sequences very playfully then I sang the "Good-bye" song and the time was up for Day 24. He laughed when he saw all the children in the kitchen when I left. He was VERY VERY happy today. This will probably normalise a bit more once the body is used to the change in medicine or awareness or neurological changes.

While I am typing this I can't help but laugh at myself... "So let me get this straight. When someone laughs a lot there must be something wrong ... either a reaction to meds or to neurological changes??? So my conclusion for today... I will enjoy his laughing and beautiful smile and not read anything in to it for now until further clarification or "NORMALISATION??" has occurred. Because you know "NORMAL" actually means you don't laugh at all, frowning sometimes seems to be more appropriate...

Dear Reader please don't be "NORMAL" today. Laugh a lot very often (not smile – LAUGH) almost like Father Christmas. Laugh from the depth of your heart, stomach and soul. You need it! Trust me. To accept a situation for what it is, you give peace permission to take your hand and intuition permission to open your eyes and see how beautiful this situation may become

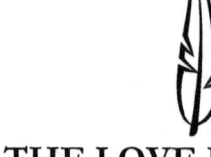

11 THE LOVE INTENTION

Day 25 – February 14, 2013

"All we need is Love..." got stuck in my head, the moment I lifted myself up from the bed to. Nooooooo! Now I will probably be singing that specific sentence the whole day. Probably you will too.

It is Valentine's Day. Today doesn't necessarily have to be aimed at a specific person, but rather at that specific feeling. A feeling so powerful it has been known to have crippled empires, healed the impossible and done the amazingly unthinkable.

Without love the world would be very bland and colourless. Harry Frederick Harlow's (October 31, 1905 – December 6, 1981) controversial (or cruel) studies have given humans necessary insight into the effect that isolation from society and lack of love has on infant monkeys. Quite frankly, I still don't understand why that was necessary since love- deprived people and children are widely spread and the effect of love-deprivation is very well known. Nothing on this planet is meant to experience "lovelessness".

Another highly controversial and much-criticised study was done by Dr. Masaru Emoto, when he exposed water to different emotions and then froze the water to study the crystal formations. The crystals of the water that was exposed to negative talk and hate were distorted, while the crystals of the water exposed to love and positive words where beautifully formed.

Although a lot of critics question his methods and scientific approach I think it is definitely something to consider as we as human consist of 70% water. What a frightening thought.

"Love changes everything", played on the radio while driving to Gabriella Centre. Very suitable for Valentine's Day, I thought, and so true. At the Centre everything was peaceful and calm. Jamie was fully alert when he entered the room. He looked a bit hyper or restless. I knew from the look of things, today must be a very relaxing day.

After sequence 1, I did a slow tapping sequence. I then used a massage technique where, using my whole hand put pressure on his skin and then released it slowly. We started with the head and then moved to the shoulders, back, chest, sides, arms, hips, legs and feet. I worked very carefully and slowly because I decided that there would be no seizures in today's session. I then did another tapping sequence on emotional release (fear, confusion, anger).

The foot massage followed where I targeted certain acupressure points on the soles of the feet. One of the nurses suddenly burst into the room by accident and I got quite a fright. Jamie started laughing and he laughed and laughed and laughed. I wasn't sure why he laughed. Was he laughing at me, did he get a fright, was this an emotional release or was it another seizure?

After the session I watched the video footage and still I couldn't see any indication of a seizure. Mmmmm... You are one interesting boy Mister Jamie.

It must be very hard for him... Every time something good or bad happens whether he is lifting his arm, bending his leg or laughing he is being second guessed and needs to prove it is not a seizure. Today, I have consciously decided that I will never do that again – that is second guess you Mister Jamie.

It is, as it is. After the feet I did another tapping sequence, and then I started the same massage again. Last but not least I did a tapping sequence. We did four very lengthy tapping sequences today in one session, without a seizure. WOW!

With all this emotional release going on especially on Valentine's Day, it reminded me of Lao Tzu: "If you are depressed you are living in the past. If you are anxious you are living in the future. If you are at peace you are living in the present."

Day 26 – February 15, 2013

"Consult not your fears but your hopes and your dreams. Think not about your frustrations, but about your unfulfilled potential. Concern yourself not with what you tried and failed in, but with what it is still possible for you to do." - Pope John XXIII

Jamie was asleep today when I arrived. I gently picked him up and carefully placed him on the mat. He was sleeping very peacefully – no snoring, just real deep breathing. I quickly started with sequence 1 and then started with the first of three tapping sequences. While he was sleeping I did as much tapping as possible. His body was very relaxed after the third tapping sequence.

After the tapping sequences he started to cough and kept on coughing for one and a half minutes. Then he was awake and alert and his eyes were wide open. Those beautiful chocolate eyes... staring at me and at the pictures on the wall. His eyes looked very wise eyes. It seemed as if they had seen the world and all its wisdom.

I then moved to the massage of the feet. His legs were stubborn and strong today, I had difficulty bending them. I did another sequence on the lungs (again) to clear the phlegm.

He had so much heartburn and what seemed like reflux today. "I hope the probiotics will kick in before it starts to burn his throat," I thought. I then decided to tap on it with him. This was our 5th tapping sequence for today's session (The most tapping sequences we have done so far in a session over the past 26 days).

Sixty minutes raced past today and am not even sure where it all went. All I know is we had no fits or any "erratic" behaviour (laughing, crying or screaming) during today's session. Just a very awake and aware Mister Jamie. Well done!

"Today is a new day, all is well, everything is okay and I am safe"

Day 27 – February 16, 2013

As the security gate closed behind me, my tears started streaming down my face. I saw in my rear view mirror our cat following my car all the way up to the garage. I silently smiled through my tears. She is such a special creature. The past 27 days have been filled with ups and downs (such is life). I think I probably had a feeling Day 27 was going to be a tougher day. I got up early this morning and started tapping on letting go of the control button and trusting in the process of life...
A sore sight greeted me this morning. Jamie had an accident somewhere yesterday and bumped his mouth. One of his front teeth was knocked forward and was a blue blackish colour. The gum surrounding the tooth seemed painful. "EINA!!", as we would say in Afrikaans – meaning ouch.

He was awake and peaceful when I picked him up and placed him on the mat. After sequence 1, I did a quick tapping sequence on the discomfort in the mouth – I was sure that there must be some sort of discomfort. I told him about my little girl who bumped her head twice last night against the same chair and how the bruise is bragging on her forehead this morning. "You kids are really keeping us, the parents, on our knees," I told him laughingly.

We look at a new-born baby promising ourselves that we will take care of them, protect them and teach them all the important lessons we wished we knew when we were small. Then we realize there aren't enough sponges in the world to put around them to protect them, we can only teach them to be positive, respect and love life, enjoy the now and be grateful.

The most important lesson is actually for us, as parents, to trust in the process of life. Our children need to learn their own lessons. All we can do, as parents, is to support them regardless of what choices they have made and which experiences they welcome into their lives.

I then did a synchronization exercise and started a visualization of muscle, nerves and cells connecting and communicating. After that we did a tapping sequence integrating all the processes that we have tapped on and all the exercises we have done. This sequence lasted 15 minutes – and guess what?

NO SEIZURE! Wow... There were no seizures during yesterday or today's sessions. Today's session took 58 minutes. I picked Jamie up, sang the "Good-bye" song and placed him back into his chair. His neck fell forward. As if he had forgotten that he doesn't really use his neck, he picked up his head and stared out of the window. I stood quietly watching him.

A noise outside the door brought him back to awareness and his head fell back. I was ecstatic! It reminded me of when a baby learns to stand. They will pull themselves up against couches or chairs and then stand. One day they will be lost in thought and let go of the couch, but still stand. Once they become aware of what is happening they will quickly grab the couch or fall to the floor.
This will happen until their confidence has increased and they have dared to try it alone more often.

With lots of praise I asked him to lift his arm so I could put the tray back ... and he did just that. Thank you, Mister Jamie...

Walking up the stairs of our house the tears were still streaming.
My husband gave me a big hug and I told him what happened to Jamie's tooth and everything that happened in the session. Very solemnly he said: "It just goes to show how much can happen in 30 days." I started to laugh. "Yes, exactly just that."

Closing thought...

"I am open and receptive to all the wonderful things life has in store for me and I welcome all positive change. I am safe to stand up and welcome healing and growing. All is well, and I am safe."

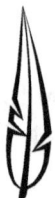

12 WHO WAS THE HERO?

Day 28 – February 17, 2013

As always, Sunday morning started very peaceful and serene. I quickly got up and dressed, made breakfast for the kids and off I went. My little one tried to negotiate a deal, on my way out, to come with me, but my husband conjured up a quick game and stole all the attention (he is such an angel). Tough morning for him though, because he has to get them and himself ready and "girlie"-up their hair, so that they are ready to go to church when I get back.

Arriving at Gabriella Centre, the quiet atmosphere smiled at me from the inside. I could hear a radio playing softly somewhere. Jamie was just getting ready when I arrived. He looked a bit hyper. Eyes looking left and right, breathing a bit fast. Oh dear, one of those days...

When I picked him out of his chair, I suddenly noticed he was assisting me and it was quite easy to pick him up. He felt stronger and not just "hanging" anymore. I smiled on the inside. During the first half of the session it seemed as if he had a few cramps. His legs would go up and down as if he was running. After sequence 1 we did leg exercises. I asked him to push my hand away and he did. His legs were really getting strong. We did a few more exercises and suddenly the "S"-word happened again. It looked painful and lasted 15 seconds. Afterwards he was wide awake. I started a tapping sequence on his left hand. I combined the tapping sequence with massage. I then moved to his right hand. After the second tapping sequence he started to cough and I had to put him back on the pillow. I quickly calmed his breathing and his heart beat slowed down. He completely calmed down. After a grounding exercise, I massaged the feet.

Then I started with the third tapping sequence. This tapping sequence was very important: "I lovingly declare that I release all the resistance to heal." The tapping sequence lasted 15 minutes. He calmed down completely. There were no seizures during this sequence. I then held him upright and we exercised the neck muscles. We sang the "Good-bye" song and I picked him up and placed him in his chair.

His head fell forward. I asked him to lift up his head. I could clearly see how he was trying. The head rest was blocking the side and he couldn't yet roll his head to the other side and bring his head up. The important fact is: learning is happening and motor pathways are forming. He wasn't smothering himself while his head was hanging and he breathed easily. The same patience we have with a baby's development will be needed.

Jamie was very happy and friendly when I pushed him into the kitchen. It was almost as if he was bragging with his performance. I was happy that he was peaceful and calm. Just like a baby... the same motor development stages must be taught to remind him and confidence in himself must be built. It might take a shorter time or maybe a little longer, but he has comprehension and learning is happening....

Jamie is truly an inspiration and his potential is unlimited.
When I arrived at my house the kids and my husband looked polished and were ready to go. My thoughts were with a little boy with chocolate-brown eyes and a will bigger than Table Mountain.

Reflecting on the past few days, I became aware of a thought that was jumping up and down in my head. "Who is saving who, Tanya De Villiers?"

Day 29 – February 18, 2013

"If I want to be loved as I am, then I need to be willing to love others as they are." – Louise Hay

The too familiar feeling of a dry mouth has returned this morning. The roads were quiet on this Monday and I was at Gabriella Centre in literally three minutes. Strange how when you want something to take longer, it usually rushes past even faster. I wanted to savour every minute of this morning.

Jamie was wide awake when the nurse brought him to me in the room. She carried him because they had to change something on his chair. I took him and placed him on the mat. Like yesterday and the day before he seemed a bit anxious.

I focused on my breathing and heartbeat to slow his down while proceeding with sequence 1. "In the midst of movement and chaos, keep stillness inside of you." The words of Deepak Chopra, echoed in my mind. I realised my anxiousness was directly affecting Jamie. Children are like that you know. Little sponges... they will take your emotions, filter them and absorb them. You might feel some sort of relief, but they are the ones who are now burdened with you emotions. Very unfair!

As parents, we always try to protect them from all the bad there is in the world, not realising how much fear, anxiety, self-doubt and anger they have already encountered just by trying to be close to the people they love. The lies we try to tell ourselves are seen and engraved in their little beings, by the ones we think are still too young to understand.

"I've learned that people will forget what you said, people will forget what you did, but people will never forget how you made them feel."- Maya Angelou

I used a dummy to try to stimulate the sucking reflex. He chewed on the dummy and then spat it out. After the third time (of spitting the dummy out), I tried to put it back and he placed his tongue in the mouth opening and I couldn't get it in. "Is a dummy not good for your image, Mister Jamie?" I laughingly said.

We moved on to the first tapping sequence on the hands, while massaging them. I then moved to the legs and feet. I asked him to wiggle his legs and "Eureka!" he did. Not only once but a few times.

In the second tapping sequence I focused on neck muscles and the mouth. I then placed him on my lap and did the neck exercises. When the neck was up, he had no trouble moving it from left to right. To keep the neck up was another story, but this too would come. He has made immense progress in the past 29 days.

I placed him on the mat again. The last tapping sequence of this session was used to facilitate the integration of all the tapping that had happened so far. I sang the "Good-bye" song and finished with a grounding exercise.

The nurse brought the chair back and I picked him up and placed him in it. His head fell forward again. Unlike yesterday, he lifted his head and his eyes lifted and looked at me. He gave a deep breath and used the movement of the chest to lift his head completely. I praised him. "Well done Mister Jamie, Well done."

He is getting stronger and smarter every day. I asked the nurses not to pick his head up when it falls forward. They can only help when he is struggling to breath. He can do it on his own. "I trust in the process of life and I am safe."

Day 30 – February 19, 2013

"The man who acquires the ability to take full possession of his own mind may take possession of anything else to which he is justly entitled." - Andrew Carnegie

This day has arrived... I felt fluey when I got up this morning. Instinctively I knew it had nothing to do with allergies or radical weather patterns. It was directly linked to my anxiety that Day 30 has arrived and the uncertainty of what is going to happen afterwards. In a way, I was angry that I hadn't made it 40 days, seeing that 40 days are linked to "renewing" in so many cultures.

After my own morning Tapping session, I realised that this was never just a 30- day project. It was, maybe, for me but when it comes to a child, a parent's work is never done. Not even when they are grown up. Jamie's mother is starting tomorrow with me, to see and learn what I am doing with him. She will then take over the process when the time is right. I am so grateful that she is willing. In a way I know his development will improve very quickly with his mother, because a mother has an intuition that no other can compare to.

When I climbed into my car to take my daughter to school, I deliberately decide to have no emotion about Day 30 until it was done. We laughed and talked about horses all the way to school. I told her about a wonderful lady I met yesterday who was doing EFT on horses. My five- year old laughed and asked: "how does she get them to stand still?" She carried on asking all sorts of questions which I will have to Google before she comes home today. How far can a horse run? How fast can a horse run? What do they eat? How many teeth do they have?

Etc. This conversation was a very good distraction (and very amusing).

Before I pushed the button at the Gabriella Centre, I took a deep breath and reminded myself: "I trust in the process of life, all is well, everything is okay and I am safe." The nurse opened the gate with a huge smile and a friendly hello. She quickly took him to the changing room while I again reminded the nurses not to assist Jamie when his head falls forward unless he can't breathe. I noticed Jamie's tooth was out and asked him if he is expecting the Tooth Fairy. He smiled as if he understood what I was saying.

The nurse brought Jamie to the room after they had finished changing his nappy. He was quiet. I picked him up from the chair and placed him on the mat. We quickly started the session, as usual, with our starting prayer. I then placed the dummy in his mouth and started tapping. This was the first of three very lengthy sequences. Each sequence lasted 15 to 20 minutes. I didn't substitute the face tapping with hand tapping. It was the "full Monty". These tapping sequences were directly related to my conversation with Sandra Pedegana, from Free To Be You, yesterday. She commented that I should maybe try Matrix Re-imprinting and I thought it was a great idea. The only reservation I had was: I have never done it before.

I would, however, be attending a course in March and the founder Karl Dawson would be presenting it, but the future course didn't mean anything to me at that moment. I then thought back at the words of Liesel Teversham, "you can't do anything wrong with tapping as long as your intention is pure and directed at healing." The body knows, I reminded myself.

With a deep breath I started the process. I tapped on 15-month- old Jamie, using visualisation, while tapping on the five- year old Jamie. We tapped on the very high fever and the chaos that surrounded him. I told him everything was going to be okay, even though there were a lot of people surrounding him, saying he was going to die and he would never make it.

We tapped on the emotions of suddenly being alone, on the seizure that happened because of the fever. I assured him the fever was gone and he was safe. We kept on tapping on all the negative things that 15-month-old Jamie all the way to five-year old Jamie must have heard and probably almost believed and we cleared that. I tapped on the support of healthy cells and muscle memories and I recalled it from the 14-month- old Jamie. The first EFT session was 20 minutes. He then spat the dummy out.

I then did a brief hand massage and started with the second sequence, going through different memories. I placed the dummy back in his mouth. After another 20- minute session I started with a brief foot and leg massage.

The dummy was again taken out of his mouth. He was completely relaxed. He started to make the snoring noise and I reminded him to breathe normally and he did. We then did the third and final tapping sequence. This time I said nothing. I just repeatedly thought the body knows what was needed now. This session was 15 minutes. He had no seizures during today's session.

After the "Good-bye" song, I picked him up and placed him in his chair. He head fell forward and I showed him how he could roll his head so that it was upright. We practised it four times. Today's session was one hour and 20 minutes. He was very peaceful and calm.

It has been a great 30 days. I can't believe how much this little five- year-old boy has taught me. He taught me gratitude, he taught me that there was never a reason to give up even when circumstances seemed to make it all impossible. He showed me that even when pain was unbearable one could still manage to smile. I was shown that to accept the "now" for what it is, is a greater strength than to be wishing for something else. Out of acceptance and peace, miracles are born. And, most importantly, I learned that "Life isn't happening to you, it is responding to you."

I thought long and hard and even procrastinated a bit before I forced myself just to sit down and start writing. I have more than 30 hours' worth of footage showing how Jamie could comprehend certain tasks that I had set out for him, showing how he was trying to help and exercise his muscles. It shows how he could show emotion that was not just linked to seizures or cramps.

It clearly shows that he could recognise people and definitely knew when his mother was in the room. The footage has shown that he responded well to games and songs and he could even focus when he looked at a page in a story book. There were dramatic changes in his awareness and his response to noises and sounds, even turning his head towards the sounds.

The ability to move muscles at specific times when asked to was amazing. He lifted his hands, wiggled his legs, wiggled his toes, tried to lift his neck, laughed when being tickled. His general health increased even though we had to clear the phlegm every now and again. I suspect the phlegm is produced because of acidity levels and might be linked to his milk.

He started to cough successfully and was able to clear the phlegm from his lungs and vocal cords. He sneezed a few times, which had never happened before. His gagging reflex has returned. Frequency in arm and leg movements has increased. I have concluded that he can comprehend and perform certain instructions such as lift your hands, wiggle your toes, wiggle your legs, lift up your head and "say" hello.

His interaction with people improved. This included touching hands, smiling when being spoken to and turning his neck and eyes towards the person interacting. His general state of awareness increased dramatically. His seizures became less.

He is a beautiful boy with so much to give. It is crucial that he gets stimulation and love as much as possible. This will expedite the process and increase the retention of the new processes that have been implemented. Muscle activity will prohibit loss of receptors. If activity seize it will disassemble synapses as proven by Research led by Jeff W. Lichtman, M.D., Ph.D., at Washington University School of Medicine in St. Louis. (Science, October 15, 1999.)

It has been determined that he can swallow and small amounts of porridge or pumpkin can be given to him. His epilepsy medicine has been decreased by 5ml per dosage (which is given three times a day). He has been on this medicine since he was 18 months old. The seizures have made radical curves from almost nothing to huge ones and then stabilized. I think it is the body's way of re-establishing balance.

I have found that since his dosage has been adjusted his state of awareness has increased dramatically. This, in turn, has directly impacted his responses to sensory stimuli and then, unfortunately, for the first week after the alteration in dosage it was a battlefield with his seizures. The changes in severity of his seizures, however, have become less radical and they seem to be stabilizing. I have to monitor the dosage for the next few weeks so that the body can find a balance and then hopefully (over a longer period) the medicine can be altered again. This alteration has been done under the supervision of his paediatrician.

His mother's biggest observation was on his the functionality and his ability to focus for longer periods of time. She also noticed that he would cough when she asked him to say hello. I am hopeful for him and his family and thankful for the journey...

This little boy with a huge will to reach out and great determination has opened my eyes in so many ways. I showed his parents how to tap and suggested activities to do over the next week. I enjoyed seeing the family interact with him and I knew, just as the brain fights for balance, so do we, as human beings, also fight to normalise life.

Saving a trapped Angel... -Tanya De Villiers

I stared deep into your dark eyes
O, seemingly lost soul,
Seeking answer, I felt was needed to know

But, I was wrong... You weren't lost
Not lost, at all – and the answers were apparent
Not meant for you, but for us.

I tried to free this perceived trapped angel-
From a cage, only created by our own minds...

But I failed... For I cannot unlock an open gate.

I reached into the depths of my heart,
Trying to hear your helpless pleas...

But I couldn't... your peaceful smile silenced my frantic voices-
The warmth of your presence calmed the storms
The peaceful silence led me to higher ground.

I charged in like a brave soldier-
Only to find there was nothing to fear, nothing to fight

My bravery seemed insignificant to your courage.

I came to free a trapped angel...
Only to find the trapped one was me-
Thank you little angel, for setting me free.

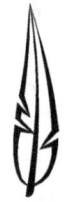

13   THE JOURNEY ONLY STARTED

"In the depth of winter, I finally learned that within me there
lay an invincible summer."
— Albert Camus

Within the next two weeks I was invited to be a guest and
helper at EFT training level 1 and 2 and I received a
sponsorship to attend the Matrix Re-imprinting training with
Karl Dawson and Caryl Westmore (this time the sponsorship
was for real). During this time I developed laryngitis and a
weird cough that would come and go as it pleased.

Feeling under the weather I drove, in the early hours of the
morning, to Cape Town. It was a perfect day, with less than
perfect traffic. I was greeted by more than 40 flamingos in
flight. With their pink feathers and the black stripes visible at
the end of the wings, they flew in graceful synchronisation. It
was an amazing sight. The wild ducks were also in flight and I
couldn't help but wonder if the end of the season was on its
way...

I arrived very early and waited for the rest of the delegates to arrive. One by one they did. It was fantastic to be surrounded by wonderful like-minded people. People whom I felt I have known all of my life. For the second time this year it felt as if I was exactly where I was supposed to be.

During the week we had many opportunities to work/practice EFT on each other and many opportunities to go on stage and sit as volunteers. To me that was very strange and I felt somewhat perplexed. "People actually volunteered to talk about their feeling in front of so many people?" The word weird came to mind a couple of times.

As children in a South African culture, we were often taught that you do not walk with your feelings on your sleeve and if you can't say anything positive it is better to keep quiet. (Or at least that was part of my up-bringing and my family's culture...). This meant that I never went on stage during the week of training and I very rarely had someone work with me in group sessions. I was therefore quick off the mark, volunteering to do EFT on someone else.

If there was enough time in the group sessions and I was obliged to be the volunteer, I would instantly start to cough. We would stop and only carry on once the cough had subsided. The cough was very frustrating, it felt as if everyone started to realise that it was emotion causing this cough.

Karl Dawson followed me outside, while we had a short break and asked me if I have noticed that I would start to cough when emotion started to build up. Feeling very embarrassed, I nodded in agreement. "Great, now everyone knew!" I thought.

Every time I would start to cough, I would think everyone knew I am getting emotional, then I would feel embarrass and the cough would only get worse. It was very stressful. That specific evening, when arriving home I fell into my husband's arms and sobbed. The mere thought of falling apart in front of strangers was horrific. What were they thinking? Why won't this darned cough just go away? Can't a cough be just a cough? – I asked him... But, we both weren't fooled and we knew the truth. Tomorrow was the last day and I will face it with this fool's courage I thought I had – "Just get it over and done Tanya."- I softly said to myself.

I felt like a bird with ruffled feathers when I got up the morning of the last training day. I didn't even put on make-up and I wore sneakers with my denim (this very rarely happens). At least I will feel comfortable in this discomfort. Although I was happy this emotional torment would be coming to an end, it was sad to think that some of these people I am not going to see again.

Wonderful enlightened beings of wonder and hope. At the end of the week we have all seen each other's dark side and secrets, and still there were no rejection. There were only hope and healing. In a way I was angry that I sabotaged my own healing and prolonged my suffering. "Why do you do that Tanya?" I angrily asked while driving to the venue.

Caryl Westmore had an opportunity to facilitate the last section of the Matrix- Re-imprinting course. She asked for a volunteer. "Someone who wanted to write a book, but experienced some blocks or self-sabotage." My heart began to race. For the past sixteen years, writing a book was one of my much longed for goals. I would start to write a book and then discard it. Nothing was ever good enough to keep on writing.

Almost everyone's hand shot up. In my heart I really wanted to volunteer, but seeing all the hands I thought that it wouldn't happen. I mean...My laryngitis hadn't gone yet and my cough had got worse as the week progressed. Not to mention that I was sitting right at the back where no one ever looks, or so I thought. Everything in me urged me to put my hand up and then I did.

I was so hoping she would pick me but I dreaded going up on stage. She went through the whole room. One by one she asked every person whose hand was up, to tell her more. Then she would say: "No, I need a specific belief." or "Maybe, let's hear if there is someone else." It seemed as if she was looking for something specific and I wasn't sure what it was. Finally she came to me. I can't even remember what I said or what she asked, but she picked me. As I approached the stairs I immediately started to cough. I could feel how the stress and tension in my body were building up.

She asked me where I think this writer's block originated from. The first memory that came up was when I wanted to publish my poetry book and university and one of the Professors told me that there wasn't a market for poetry books and it will only cost me money. He also continued to say that one of my personal favourite poems didn't make any sense. I threw my journal away and gave up the idea almost instantly.

She asked me if there were an earlier memory that can be associated with this block. While she tapped on my head I suddenly remember a very vague memory of my father telling me when I was three years old, that I shouldn't be so emotional. The memory was very vague but the feelings were clear. I was crying about something – nothing significant now, but it meant something then.

My dad probably got tired of the dramatic weeping and in the chaos and drama it felt to me, as three year old Tanya, that he actually said that it is wrong to be emotional. We cleared the emotions in the memory with Matrix Re-Imprinting, of three year old Tanya and then cleared the emotions of the University Tanya. She did an exercise where I was to imagine myself as a writer in the Matrix and visualise the books I have written. In a very short space of time we managed to sort out the hindrances of completing the book but we also got to the bottom of what caused me to lose my voice.

I created a limiting belief that it was silly to express my emotions. The effect of this limiting belief was that every time I would get emotional something that felt like a big block would sit in my throat and prevent me from expressing myself clearly. This meant that I would actually start to cough when finding myself in an uncomfortable position.

The book that I had been trying to write for years was always postponed for some reason or the other. One book would be started with great vigour and a while later, I would think it to be silly and start a new one. Carol continued with a matrix re-imprinting session and almost instantaneously my cough disappeared. The next day my voice returned and I felt free.

Over the next couple of days I had a dramatic surge of creativity. It wasn't long after the course when my family and I decided to have an impromptu holiday in Vereeniging, the city from where we'd moved. The visit was marvellous. Our younger daughter's asthma subsided and the children really enjoyed seeing all the grandparents. On our drive back after a very heartfelt goodbye we decided, as a family, to move back to our previous home. However, the thought of leaving Jamie, was daunting. I feared that his improvements would all be for nothing.

I saw the potential and the possibilities in us moving, but the thought of starting over again was awful. I have started over so many times in my life and frankly it wasn't getting easier. Firstly it was moving from South Africa to the UK, then moving back to South Africa when I was seven months pregnant with our first child. Then, of course, the traumatic move to Cape Town and then back to the Vaal Triangle. The difference was that this time, I felt complete peace about the move.

After the last session I had with Jamie before we moved back to Gauteng, I had a sense of finality on the way out. I looked back over my shoulder and smiled at him. It was almost as if he knew I was saying goodbye. This angel that I thought was trapped was actually freeing me. Giving me wings to fly, opening my eyes to new possibilities and reminding me that limits only exist for those believing in them.

My prayer as I climbed into the car was; "God please send him an angel to guide him on his path, a comfortable hug to fill his heart, an ear that recognises your voice, the ability to block out the negatives and a will that believes when no one else does. Let his heart speak to many. Grant him peace and unconditional love, Amen."

"Spring passes and one remembers one's innocence.
Summer passes and one remembers one's exuberance.
Autumn passes and one remembers one's reverence.
Winter passes and one remembers one's perseverance."

— Yoko Ono

Tanya De Villiers

APPENDICES

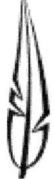

Appendix 1

What is Kinder-kinetics?

It is a scientifically based program that focusses on children's motor development and milestones through movement. The goal and objective of Kinder-kinetics is correct and improve motor and physical development of children with a fun and playful activity program that facilitate development.

Kinder-kinetics aims in helping to develop children holistically by stimulating, remedying & promoting specific motor & physical movement. The specific focus of Kinder-kinetics is targeting to evaluate a child's gross motor skills with specific test batteries. Each session strives to incorporate the fun factor with the use of creative equipment and imaginative themes.

More resources can be found at:

http://stellieskinderkinetics.wordpress.com/about/

http://www.nwu.ac.za/node/13846

http://humanities.ufs.ac.za/content.aspx?id=153

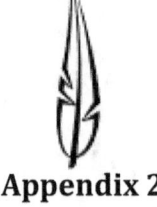

Appendix 2

What is Cerebral Palsy (CP)?

Cerebral palsy (CP) is an umbrella term denoting a group of non-contagious, non-progressive motor conditions that cause physical disability in development. Cerebral Palsy is part of a group of disabling symptoms directly linked to damage to the motor control areas of the brain. Scientific consensus still holds that CP is neither genetic nor a disease. It can be defined as a central motor dysfunction affecting muscle tone, posture and movement resulting from a permanent, non-progressive defect or lesion of the immature brain.

The symptoms may vary depending on the amount of damage to the brain and the location of damage. It can range from severe to very mild. In severe cases it can result in total inability to control bodily movements, while in mild cases a slight speech impediment can be present.

A person with Cerebral Palsy commonly exhibits other impairment, which can include: language and speech disorders, seizures, mental retardation and sensory impairments, to name a few.

Cerebral Palsy can be the result from Rubella, Rh incompatibility, birth trauma, meningitis, encephalitis, anoxia, brain hemorrhages or tumors, poisoning and other brain injuries as a result of abuse or accidents. This usually happens during prenatal, natal or postnatal. It is also understood that the vast majority of cases are congenital, coming at or about the time of birth, and/or are diagnosed at a very young age (up to 3 years) rather than during adolescence or adulthood.

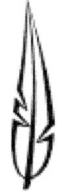

BIBLIOGRAPHY AND RESOURCES:

Websites:

http://en.wikipedia.org/wiki/Cerebral_palsy

http://www.intropsych.com/ch02_human_nervous_system/02homunc.jpg

http://kidshealth.org/kid/health_problems/brain/cerebral_palsy.html

http://www.mayoclinic.com/health/cerebral-palsy/DS00302

http://www.heartmaths.org

http://www.emofree.com

http://tanyaontapping.blogspot.com

www.eftelite.com

www.youtube.com/TanyaDeVilliers

www.matrixreimprinting.com

www.facebook.com/TanyaOnTapping

www.masaru-emoto.net/english/water-crystal.html

Books:

Bognon, L. 2004. We are here to learn. JHB: Lou Bognon

Dawson, K. & Allenby S. 2010. Matrix Reimprinting using EFT. London: Hay House

De Jager, M. 2011. Brain Development Milestones and learning. JHB: Mind Moves Institute

De Jager, M. 2009. Mind Moves: Removing Barriers to learning. Welgemoed: Metz Press

Hay, L.L. 2004. You can heal your Life. Hay House

Muccillo, A. 2008. Tapping for Kids. East Sussex: DragonRising Publishings

Teversham L. 2012. No Problem: The upside of saying no. Fish Hoek: Kima Global Publishers

Tolle, E. 2005. A New Earth: Awakening to your life's purpose. London: Penguin Books

Westmore, C. 2009. You can Break-Free Fast. Claremont: New Vision Publishing.

Winnick J.P. Adapted Physical Education and Sport. 3rd Edition. 2000

Articles:

Akaaboune M, Culican SM, Turney SG, Lichtman JW. Rapid and

reversible effects of activity on acetylcholine receptor density at the neuromuscular junction in vivo. Science, Oct. 15, 1999.

Chevalier, G. & Sinatra, S.T. Emotional Stress, Heart Rate Variability, Grounding, and Improved Autonomic Tone: Clinical Applications. Integrative Medicine Vol. 10, No. 3, Jun/Jul 2011.

Vinoth K. Ranganathan a, Vlodek Siemionowa,b, Jing Z. Liu a, Vinod Sahgal b, Guang H. Yue. From mental power to muscle power—gaining strength by using the mind. Neuropsychologia 42 (2004) 944–956.

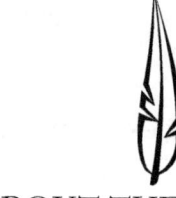

ABOUT THE AUTHOR

Tanya de Villiers was born in a small town close to the Vaal and Klip River, called Meyerton. She completes her Bachelor's degree in Human Movement Sciences and was selected to complete her Honors degree in Kinder-kinetics. In 2004 she was awarded her Master's degree in Kinder-kinetics and has published two articles in a medical journal on water activities and children with disabilities. After working in the UK as a Lecturer and therapist at different Institutions for three years, she returned back to South Africa with her husband. From 2007 to 2011 she managed to build a practice that served literally hundreds of children a month, educating them on a healthy lifestyle and optimal development through movement. In 2011 she completed a NBI course of Dr Kobus Neetling and the need for children to be optimally integrated became to her apparent. She completed the EFT level 1 and 2 course as well as the Matrix Re-imprinting standard and Advanced course. She is a great believer that children need positive reinforcement especially in their forming years from 0 up to 7. To her it has become apparent that we are not there just to educate children on right and wrong but open ourselves to be taught BY the children's deeper understanding of love. They are love and they must be loved, because only with unconditional love they and we will be formed into our true potential.

Tanya is the founder of www.eftelite.com and co-founder of Emotive Solutions Inc.

www.ingramcontent.com/pod-product-compliance
Lightning Source LLC
Chambersburg PA
CBHW070924290526
45795CB00001B/412